the**facts**

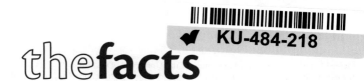

Alcoholism

FOURTH EDITION

Ann M. Manzardo PhD
Assistant Professor and Pharmacologist

Donald W. Goodwin MD
University Distinguished Professor, Emeritus

Jan L. Campbell MD
Professor of Director of Addicition Psychiatry

Elizabeth C. Penick PhD
Professor and Director of Psychology

William F. Gabrielli, Jr MD, PhD
Professor and Chair of Psychiatry
Professor of Internal Medicine

**Department of Psychiatry and Behvioral Sciences,
University of Kansas Medical center, Kansas, USA**

OXFORD
UNIVERSITY PRESS

OXFORD
UNIVERSITY PRESS

Great Clarendon Street, Oxford OX2 6DP

Oxford University Press is a department of the University of Oxford.
It furthers the University's objective of excellence in research, scholarship,
and education by publishing worldwide in

Oxford New York

Auckland Cape Town Dar es Salaam Hong Kong Karachi
Kuala Lumpur Madrid Melbourne Mexico City Nairobi
New Delhi Shanghai Taipei Toronto

With offices in

Argentina Austria Brazil Chile Czech Republic France Greece
Guatemala Hungary Italy Japan Poland Portugal Singapore
South Korea Switzerland Thailand Turkey Ukraine Vietnam

Oxford is a registered trade mark of Oxford University Press
in the UK and in certain other countries

Published in the United States
by Oxford University Press Inc., New York

© Oxford University Press 2008

The moral rights of the authors have been asserted
Database right Oxford University Press (maker)

First edition published 1981
Second edition published 1994
Third edition published 2000
Reprinted 2000, 2002, 2003, 2004 (twice), 2005, 2006
Fourth edition published 2008

British Library Cataloguing in Publication Data

Data available

Library of Congress Cataloguing in Publication Data

Data available

ISBN 978-0-19-923139-3

10 9 8 7 6 5 4 3 2 1

Typeset in Plantin
by Cepha Imaging Pvt. Ltd., Bangalore, India
Printed in China
on acid-free paper by
Asia Pacific Offset

Whilst every effort has been made to ensure that the contents of this book are as complete, accurate
and up-to-date as possible at the date of writing, Oxford University Press is not able to give any
guarantee or assurance that such is the case. Readers are urged to take appropriately qualified
medical advice in all cases. The information in this book is intended to be useful to the general
reader, but should not be used as a means of self-diagnosis or for the prescription of medication.

This book is dedicated to the late Donald W. Goodwin MD and his wife Sally. Don touched all of our lives in many different ways over many, many years as a friend, colleague, mentor, and Chair of the Department of Psychiatry and Behavioral Sciences at the University of Kansas Medical Center. His good humor, his modesty, his vast knowledge of alcoholism, and his remarkable ability to focus on essentials without getting lost in trivia remain, even today, important lessons for us all.

Preface to the fourth edition

It has been nearly a decade since the death of Donald W. Goodwin, the original author of *The Facts* series on alcoholism and co-author of the current work. The third edition was the last original work from Donald Goodwin and still today stands as an honest accurate commentary on the devastating nature of this disease as well as the unique challenges it presents to researchers, health-care providers, affected individuals and their families. Donald was a world-renowned expert and a pioneer in alcoholism research. He helped the world to focus on the importance of genetics and family history in the development of alcoholism. As a psychiatrist, distinguished professor, journalist, and novelist, Donald Goodwin had a special gift for language. His words captured the very essence of alcoholism ... from the perspective of the scientist and the eyes of the drinker. He always knew just the right quote to capture the heart, soul, and genuine suffering associated with this disease. Donald Goodwin knew his facts on alcoholism, and the information in his books was spot on accurate ... for its time. But considerable time has passed since his death and some things have now changed. *The facts* are due for an update and we, his followers at the University of Kansas Medical Center, have tried to carry on his tradition.

In the years since Donald Goodwin's death in 1999, we have seen an explosion of new technologies available for the study of the brain and behavior. These technologies have given scientists and clinicians the opportunity to 'look inside' and better understand the brains of people who drink. These advances offer dramatic changes for research on alcoholism. They may open the door to the development of useful treatment strategies designed to help recovering alcoholics resist the powerful urges to drink again. The fourth edition benefits from some of these nascent advances and comments upon the nature of the disease and strategies for treatment. Although we continue to use the term 'alcoholism' in this book—that is historical. Doctors now refer to alcohol abuse and alcohol dependence, making a distinction between the two. We also save the use of the term 'alcoholic' for the same reason, but our research leads us to more properly refer to 'the person who suffers from alcohol abuse or alcohol dependence'. For now, we have retained the format of the original work and have attempted to retain much of the 'Goodwin charm'. A fifth edition will no doubt look very different.

University of Kansas Medical Center

2008

Contents

Section four
Treating alcoholism

Section 1

Alcohol

You have asked me how I feel about whiskey. All right, here is just how I stand on this question:

If when you say whiskey, you mean the devil's brew, the poison scourge, the bloody monster that defiles innocence, yea literally takes the bread from the mouths of little children; if you mean the evil drink that topples the Christian man and woman from the pinnacles of righteous, gracious living into t=he bottom-less pit of degradation and despair, shame and helplessness and hopelessness, then certainly I am against it with all of my power.

But, if when you say whiskey, you mean the oil of conversation, the philosophic wine, the stuff that is consumed when good fellows get together, that puts a song in their hearts and laughter on their lips and the warm glow of contentment in there eye; if you mean Christmas cheer; if you mean the stimulating drink that puts the spring in the old gentleman's step on a frosty morning; if you mean the drink that enables a man to magnify his joy, and his happiness, and to forget, if only for a little while, life's great tragedies and heartbreaks and sorrow; if you mean that drink, the sale of which pours into our treasuries untold millions of dollars, which are used to provide tender care for our little crippled children, our blind, our deaf, our dumb, our pitiful aged and infirmed, to build highways, hospitals and schools, then certainly I am in favor of it.

This is my stand. I will not retreat from it; I will not compromise.

Address to the legislature
by a Mississippi state senator
1958

1

Alcoholic beverages

Let us begin at the beginning: with yeast.

When yeast grows in sugar solutions without air, most of the sugar is converted (fermented) into carbon dioxide and alcohol. Carbon dioxide makes the solution bubble ('fermentation' comes from the Latin word for 'boil') and makes champagne corks pop. The alcohol is excreted. Most drinkers do not know that they are drinking yeast excrement. Would it matter?

It matters for yeast. When the alcohol concentration reaches about 12 or 13 percent, the yeast dies of acute alcohol intoxication. This is why unfortified wines, produced by fermentation alone, have alcohol concentrations of no more than 12 or 13 percent. Sherry, port, and other fortified wines have alcohol added.

As a rule, people do not drink just alcohol. They drink alcoholic beverages. Alcoholic beverages are mostly water and a two-carbon alcohol molecule called ethyl alcohol or ethanol. Tiny amounts of other chemicals, called congeners, also are present. They provide most of the taste and smell and all of the color, if any.

Because of congeners, beer can be distinguished from brandy, although both consist almost entirely of ethyl alcohol and water. Congeners, depending on the beverage, include varying amounts of amino acids, minerals, vitamins, a one-carbon alcohol called methanol or 'wood alcohol', plus the 'higher' alcohols with more than two carbons, otherwise known as fusel oil.

Even in small quantities, wood alcohol and fusel oil are poisons. So is ethyl alcohol, but a lot more of it is required to do damage. Is there enough wood alcohol and fusel oil in a cocktail to hurt anyone? Probably not, but no one is sure. To be on the safe side, some people avoid drinks with large amounts of congeners—whiskey and brandies—and drink relatively congener-free vodka. They are not aware that vodka often contains more wood alcohol—the notorious blinder[1]—than other beverages. Although there is almost certainly not enough to blind, wood alcohol does not improve vision.

Congeners vary not only from beverage to beverage but also from brand to brand, and even from bottle to bottle of the same brand. Not all brands (or bottles) of vodka contain relatively high amounts of wood alcohol, but some do. Russian vodka, the favorite of many vodka connoisseurs, sometimes contains considerable amounts of wood alcohol, although, again, not enough to be harmful.

For many years there was a movement in the USA to label alcoholic beverages as 'dangerous to your health'. Indeed they are, if taken in excess. With much opposition from the alcoholic beverage industry, Congress finally passed a law requiring a warning on alcoholic beverages that 'according to the surgeon general', women should not drink during pregnancy, nor should anyone drink who drives a car or operates machinery, followed by a warning that drinking may cause health problems. The warnings are in tiny print and often placed on bottles where they are unlikely to be seen, such as the neck. A more useful label for alcoholic beverages might list the congener content in the same way that ingredients are listed on food packages. In the small amount present in beverages, congeners may not be dangerous but heavy drinkers ingest rather a large amount of congeners, and some believe, with uncertain evidence, that some of them contribute to hangovers and medical complications from heavy drinking.

Apart from man's contribution—the brewer's art, the cosseted grape—beverages differ according to the sugar source. From grapes, wine; from grain and hops, beer; from grain and corn, whiskey; from sugar cane, rum; and originally from the lowly potato, but now mainly from grain, vodka.

Man's great achievement in improving upon yeast's modest productivity was distillation, discovered about CE 800 in Arabia ('alcohol' comes from the Arabic *alkuhl*, meaning essence). Distillation boils away alcohol from its sugar bath and re-collects it as virtually pure alcohol. Then, because pure alcohol is pure torture to drink, water is added back, so that instead of having 100 percent alcohol, you have, for example, 50 percent or 100 proof alcohol (one proof being one-half percent).

The alcohol content of most distilled alcoholic beverages is expressed in degrees of proof. This term probably developed from the seventeenth-century English custom of estimating contents by moistening gunpowder with the beverage and applying a flame to the mixture. The lowest alcohol concentration that would allow ignition—a concentration of about 57 percent alcohol by volume—was considered to be 'proof spirits'. British and Canadian regulations are still based on this yardstick; a concentration of 57.35 percent alcohol is considered to be 'proof spirits', while other concentrations are described as 'over' or 'under' proof.

In many ways, alcohol resembles water. In the body alcohol behaves like water. It travels everywhere water travels. Because of its water-like properties, ethyl alcohol can be accommodated by the body in vastly greater amounts than any other drug. A person's blood can consist of one-half percent of alcohol without producing death or even unconsciousness.

2

Alcohol in the body

→ Key points

- Alcohol in the body is normally processed rapidly by the liver; however, this process is easily overwhelmed by the consumption of large quantities of alcohol in short periods of time, and toxic levels can build up.

- Much of the harm in drinking comes from a disruption of the normal biochemical balance because of the demands of processing excessive amounts of alcohol.

- Many of the common complications of alcohol abuse result from deficiencies in essential nutrients which are common among alcoholics.

- Alcohol directly suppresses hormone production in males and females, which not only impairs sexual performance but may also alter sexual characteristics, growth, and fertility.

The metabolism of alcohol

What happens to alcohol when you drink it? Essentially the same thing that happens when you don't drink it. It turns to vinegar.

When alcohol 'sours' in the open air, bacteria are responsible. To become vinegar (acetic acid) in the body, alcohol needs two enzymes:[1] alcohol dehydrogenase and aldehyde dehydrogenase. When alcohol is broken down or 'metabolized', it is converted first to acetaldehyde (by alcohol dehydrogenase) and then to acetic acid (by acetaldehyde dehydrogenase) which can be processed and burned in place of glucose for energy. Alcohol dehydrogenase is located, in rather large supply, in the liver where the majority of alcohol processing occurs; consequently, it is the liver that suffers the most from repeated imbibing of alcohol. The second enzyme, acetaldehyde dehydrogenase, is present in abundance in all tissues. Its levels are generally sufficient to prevent the accumulation of the intermediate chemical, acetaldehyde, which is quite toxic. Acetic acid is ultimately 'burned' using the normal metabolic machinery to become carbon dioxide and water, generating 7 calories of energy per gram of alcohol in the process.

The reason that we humans have such high levels of alcohol-metabolizing enzymes in our bodies in the first place is somewhat controversial.

Did God anticipate that some day humans would develop a taste for alcohol and need a way to dispose of it? Perhaps there was another purpose.

As it turns out, these enzymes will act on any number of different alcohol and aldehyde molecules. It is widely believed that their so-called 'natural' function is, in fact, the metabolism of vitamin A which is required for healthy vision.

The harm in drinking

So what is the harm in drinking?

For your body, most of the problems start with the intake of large amounts of alcohol, quickly. Even in experienced drinkers, alcohol-metabolizing systems are easily overwhelmed, allowing alcohol to accumulate. Such drinking to drunkenness can also lead to an accumulation of acetaldehyde which can react with and damage cellular proteins and DNA. No doubt, repeated exposure to high levels of these toxins contributes to the development of many of the health problems commonly found in alcoholics.

The metabolism of alcohol also alters the normal cellular metabolic processes of the body in several specific ways.

1. There is an increase in the production of lactic acid, a cellular toxin.

2. There is an increase in uric acid which is associated with gout.

3. There is disruption of the regulation of blood sugar levels which can cause low blood sugar, especially after a night of heavy drinking.

4. There is an increase in the synthesis of fat, mainly in the liver, which can build up and clog the organ.

Such shifts in the chemical balance of the body are not usually a problem in small doses. The body is quite resilient. Over time, however, the persistent derangement of these systems can lead to serious problems.

Chronic heavy drinking can inflame the liver in particular, a condition known as alcoholic hepatitis. Hepatitis can cause cell death and permanent scarring, or cirrhosis, of the liver which can progress to death. Fortunately, cirrhosis only occurs in about 5–10 percent of alcoholics. Why only 10 percent? This is not clear, but heavy drinking appears to be the trigger in these individuals. It is clear that heavy alcohol use is damaging to many organ systems. The particular system damaged, and in whom, depends upon individual factors. Be it your liver, stomach, or pancreas, alcohol has a way of finding your weakest link. These problems are usually associated with heavy drinking, and even then may only occur in certain individuals.

Alcohol and nutrition

Alcoholics also tend to be malnourished, which only adds to their problems. Malnutrition in alcoholics can be attributed, in part, to poor dietary habits. For many alcoholics, the majority of their daily caloric intake comes from alcohol. Over time, however, the toxic effects of heavy drinking on the gut and other body systems begin to interfere with the body's ability to absorb and use dietary nutrients. In the end, the accelerated rate of alcohol processing depletes the remaining nutrient stores. This is especially true for vitamin B_1 (thiamine) which is required for the metabolism of sugars as well as alcohol. High rates of alcohol processing rob the body of thiamine, leading to deficiencies that can be severe. Severe thiamine deficiency selectively damages muscle and nerve tissues. Nerve damage in the extremities can produce neuritis, an inflammation of the peripheral nervous system. Similar damage in the brain can lead to coordination problems and memory impairments, a condition known as Wernike–Korsakoff syndrome. A large number of the adverse health effects found with heavy drinking are actually due to alcoholism-related nutritional deficiencies and not to the alcohol itself. We will review these conditions in Chapter 6.

Alcohol, sex, and hormones

Alcohol's effects on the libido and sexual performance are legendary. Some of these effects are due to alcohol's potent inhibitory actions on testosterone production in men and estrogen release in women. One study reported a 40 percent decrease in blood testosterone levels among college-age men after a single heavy-drinking episode. Alcohol disrupts hormone production at all levels of the endocrine system, beginning in the brain. Alcohol interferes not only with sexual performance but also with sexual characteristics in general, including fertility. Therefore, men who think that drinking alcohol will 'make a man' of them have got it backwards.

Frequent short-term decreases in testosterone levels caused by heavy drinking can permanently alter certain hormone responses in the brain, disrupt muscle and prostate function, and interfere with the formation of bone, leading to osteoporosis. These effects appear to be amplified in males exposed to repeated drops in testosterone or permanent hypogonadism[2] in adolescence.

In females, similar effects on estrogen production can disrupt the normal menstrual cycle and reproductive functions. Alcohol abuse in younger women and girls may alter bone growth and fertility. The abuse of alcohol in older women can produce osteoporosis and trigger the onset of menopause.

3

Alcohol and its effects

> **→ Key points**
>
> ◆ The effects of most drugs, including alcohol, depend upon the amount and rate at which the drug is absorbed into the bloodstream.
>
> ◆ Heavy drinking for long periods of time can lead to tolerance to the effects of alcohol.
>
> ◆ The phases of intoxication may or may not be accompanied by shifts in the emotional state of the drinker.

The effects of any drug depend on the dose. The chance of death occurring from a sip of beer is remote. A quart of whiskey drunk in an hour will kill most men. This dose–effect rule applies to any substance that a person consumes. Everything is either a poison or harmless depending on the dose. People die from drinking too little water and from drinking too much. Of course, quantity is not everything. To the amount consumed must be added other factors that influence a drug's effects

Blood alcohol concentrations

It is not really how much alcohol a person drinks that determines their level of intoxication but, rather, how much gets into their bloodstream. The rate of increase in blood alcohol levels is also an important factor; in general, the faster the rate of absorption, the more striking the effect. The alcoholic may attempt to maximize the rate of alcohol absorption by selecting a higher-potency beverage, drinking on an empty stomach, or drinking large quantities at once.

Some alcohol is absorbed through the stomach wall, but most reaches the bloodstream through the small intestine. To maximize absorption, alcohol must reach the small intestine in the highest possible concentration and the shortest possible time. Both the size and the contents of the stomach factor into this equation. People who have had gastric bypass surgery to reduce the size of their stomachs to help them lose weight find that they get drunk faster than previously. In a study prompted by an episode of *Oprah*,[1] researchers found that subjects who had obesity surgery achieved blood alcohol levels three times higher than normal control subjects—presumably because of a dramatic enhancement of alcohol absorption. This effect has caused some to wonder whether gastric bypass surgery may increase the risk of alcohol problems in some people.

The presence or absence of food in the stomach and the type of beverage consumed will hasten or retard alcohol absorption. Food in the stomach acts like a sponge that soaks up the brew and will delay absorption into the bloodstream. The type of beverage consumed can also influence the rate at which the alcohol is absorbed. Alcohol in the form of different beverages was given to subjects with and without food. Although the same amount of alcohol was consumed over the same length of time, the blood-alcohol concentration varied greatly. Gin on an empty stomach produced peak blood-alcohol levels far greater than beer combined with a meal.

This is not meant to suggest that the type of alcohol consumed has anything to do with the likelihood of becoming an alcoholic. Alcohol is alcohol. One can become an alcoholic just as easily drinking beer as whiskey or gin. It's a matter of timing and quantity.

There has been speculation about why alcoholism rates in France and Italy differ so much. Italy, with the lower rate, has a national tradition of drinking wine mainly with meals, while the French tend to drink wine between meals as well as with them. When wine and pasta compete for transport across the intestinal wall, it is not surprising that pasta, finishing the race first, will prevent the wine from making much headway.

Mixing food and alcohol also produces a slight increase in the oxidation of alcohol and hence its removal from the bloodstream. This may partly explain the lower blood-alcohol level when food and alcohol are combined. It may also partly explain the known reluctance of alcoholics to eat while drinking, since presumably the alcoholic has no strong desire to remove alcohol from his bloodstream any faster than necessary.

Tolerance

As people drink more over days, months, and years, they gradually need to drink more and more to obtain the same effect. This physical adaptation is called tolerance. Its importance is often exaggerated. A seasoned alcoholic at the prime of his drinking capacity may be able to drink, at most, twice as much as a teetotaler of similar age and health. Compared with tolerance for morphine, which can be manifold, tolerance for alcohol is modest. (Apparently, alcohol in the same amount is as lethal for heavy drinkers as for light drinkers, although the experimental studies required to prove this have not been done for obvious reasons. Tolerance to opiates, including morphine and heroin, far surpasses levels lethal to non-users.)

More striking than 'acquired' tolerance may be inborn tolerance. Individuals vary widely in the amount of alcohol that they can naturally tolerate. Some people, no matter how hard they might try, cannot drink more than a small amount of alcohol without developing a headache, upset stomach, or dizziness. They rarely become alcoholics, but deserve no credit for it. Their 'alcohol problem' is that they cannot drink very much.

Other people are able to drink large amounts with hardly any ill effects. They seem to have been born with a capacity to tolerate alcohol in large amounts and did not develop it entirely from practice. They can become alcoholics, and some do.

Difference in tolerance to alcohol applies not only to individuals but also to racial groups. For example, many people of Asian descent develop flushing of the skin, sometimes with nausea, after drinking only a little alcohol. This is uncomfortable and may explain why alcoholism is rare in these groups. Native Americans are also said to be intolerant to alcohol, but the nature of the intolerance is more ambiguous and does not appear to discourage heavy drinking.

Mind-set and setting

Any drug response that affects thinking and mood is bound to be influenced by expectation. Alcohol is no exception. If a person believes that alcohol will improve his mood, diminish fatigue, make him feel sexy, or have salutary effects, the chances that these pleasant changes will occur may be improved. The same goes for expectations of unpleasant changes.

In medicine this is called the placebo effect: drugs tend to do for people what they expect them to do. The placebo effect presumably has little or no role in the treatment of pneumonia with antibiotics—although one cannot be certain—but it has powerful implications for the treatment of psychiatric disorders. Sometimes sugar pills help psychiatric disorders almost as much as expensive and potentially toxic tranquillizers or antidepressants.

It is the gap between the sugar pill's performance and that of the 'active' drug that justifies the prescription of the drug. Sometimes that gap is surprisingly small. Placebos can even produce side-effect-like symptoms such as head-aches, nausea, and rash. Everyone is slightly susceptible to suggestion, and some more than others.

It is difficult to know how much the effect of alcohol in any given person on any particular occasion is influenced by expectation or mind-set. Presumably, the stronger the dose the smaller is the placebo effect. However, it is a common laboratory and social observation that some people get 'drunk' on very little alcohol. This may be because they want or expect to get drunk quickly.

However, mind-set refers to more than expectation. If a person is tired, alco-hol may have more of an antifatigue effect than usual. If he is hungry, it may make him more hungry (or less). If his mood is good, it may become better. If bad, worse. All of this refers to mind-set—the psychological and physical state of the person at the time he proceeds to drink.

Mind-set, to a considerable extent, is linked to setting. Where is the person drinking? With whom? If he enjoys the people he is with, he may also enjoy the alcohol more. If the occasion is a celebration, a drink may have a livelier effect than would the same amount taken routinely before dinner.

Alcohol is said to make people talk louder, and this often seems to be true. On the other hand, two men on a deer hunt, taking a nip of scotch to warm up, may talk more quietly than usual.

The importance of mind-set and setting in shaping a person's response to alcohol should not be under-estimated, although it is difficult to study their relative influence at a given time.

The four stages of intoxication

There is an old saying that alcohol affects a person in four ways. First, he becomes jocose, then bellicose, then lachrymose, and finally comatose.

Comatose he does indeed become if he drinks enough, but the other three stages are not inevitable. Some people hardly feel jocose at all. One reason may be that they do not want to feel jocose. Their reasons for drinking may be purely social: others drink, so do they.

Many people become argumentative when they drink and some combative, but these responses are strongly influenced by social circumstances and personality. Countless parties are held nightly in middle-class suburbia and, although drinking is common, fighting is not.

This is not to deny that drinking may bring out the beast in man. Alcohol is involved in at least half of all homicides in the USA, with the attacker or the victim, or both, under the influence. This probably explains why more murders occur on Saturday night than on any other evening (the fewest occur on Tuesdays). It has been suggested that one reason that fights occur in bars is that rarely are so many people thrust together so closely for such long periods, with hardly anything to do but talk, drink, and fight.

One of the paradoxes about alcohol is that people sometimes cry when they drink. Why drink then? Isn't the whole point of drinking to feel happier? The fact is, even though some people become anxious and depressed when they drink, they do not give up drinking, which challenges the widely held assumption that people drink mainly to feel less anxious and depressed. The motives for drinking, in truth, are complex and inscrutable, with no single explanation sufficing for all circumstances.

Alcohol is often described as a 'depressant' drug which depresses first the 'higher' centers in the brain and then downwardly anesthetizes the brain until finally, in lethal dosage, it snuffs out life itself by depressing the respiratory center at the base of the brain. This, like most things said about alcohol, is an over-simplification.

So what is it that alcohol is 'depressing'? Usually not activity. Most people get a 'lift' from alcohol, and many become more animated and active while drinking. Again, dosage is crucial. Alcohol in small amounts may improve certain types of performance. Apparently this is most likely to occur in activities where the person is not very proficient and where increased confidence might help. Nevertheless, in moderate to high amounts, alcohol usually diminishes performance across the board.

An interesting exception to this general rule has emerged in several studies. Apparently, if a person learns certain things, such as word lists, while intoxicated—even severely intoxicated—he will remember them better when re-intoxicated than when sober. Called 'state-dependent learning', this is one of the few exceptions to the overall impairing effect of alcohol at moderate and high dosages.

Alcohol does something else that is almost unique among drugs. It produces a classical amnesia called 'blackout'. While drinking, the drinker does highly memorable things but cannot remember them the next day. Many social drinkers have had this experience, but it occurs most frequently in alcoholics.

Myths

Some of the physical effects of alcohol should also be mentioned, if only because there are misconceptions about them.

* It is known that alcohol increases urination. It is generally not known that the increase is temporary and that after a fairly short period of drinking the need to urinate decreases. On the morning after a night of heavy drinking, a person may not urinate at all. No explanation is available.

* It is commonly believed that alcohol causes dehydration. It does not. When a person has a dry mouth and thirst after an evening of drinking, it is probably because of the astringent effect of alcohol on the mucous membranes of the mouth. If anything, heavy drinkers may be over-hydrated because of the large volume of fluid they consume.

* It is generally believed that alcohol produces a feeling of bodily warmth and therefore is just the thing for a Saint Bernard dog to carry around its neck in barrels for people to drink at a frosty football game. Alcohol produces a feeling of warmth because it dilates blood vessels in the skin. However, the warmth can be harmfully illusory. A person's resistance to the effects of severe cold, such as frostbite, is in no way increased by alcohol, although the victim may temporarily think that it is.

* It is said that some people are 'allergic' to alcohol. Members of Alcoholics Anonymous sometimes use the word 'allergy' in a metaphorical sense to explain their addiction. Alcohol is not an allergen in the usual sense. Allergens are usually proteins, while alcohol is, well, alcohol. Allergies result from an over-activity of the immune system which can also occur in response to some chemicals, including alcohol, in sensitive people, although a similar 'sensitivity' to alcohol would not result in alcoholism. Most of the physical effects of allergic reactions and chemical sensitivities (flushing, hives, breathing problems) result from the release of histamine by damaged cells. This response may explain the flushing reaction experienced by some people of Asian descent which can be prevented by antihistamine drugs. However, in this case cell damage is caused by an increase in acetaldehyde, not alcohol, in the blood because of an inherited variation in alcohol metabolism.

4

Alcohol through the ages

> ### ➲ Key points
>
> ◆ Alcohol use has been the subject of mythical lore since the earliest records of mankind.
>
> ◆ Alcohol consumption patterns have varied throughout history, but the precise incidence of alcoholism is difficult to assess for scientific as well as political reasons.
>
> ◆ Likewise, it is difficult to define a precise level of alcohol consumption which may be considered safe or 'normal'.
>
> ◆ While there appear to be clear health benefits associated with moderate alcohol use, these advantages must be tempered against ill-effects which may also appear at relatively low consumption levels.

Six millennia ago at the Sumerian trading post of Godin Tepe, in what is now western Iran, people were drinking beer and wine. In 1992, chemists identified a residue in pottery jars found in the ruins of Godin Tepe as wine or beer. The jars were all found in the same room. A scientist said, 'I think a lot of serious drinking was going on there'. The Sumerians were among the first people to develop a complex literate society of prospering city-states based on irrigation, agriculture, and widespread trade.

Beer-making began almost as soon as (or even before) people domesticated barley to make bread in the early transition by Mesopotamians to agriculture around 8000 BCE. A long-standing debate in archeology centers on the question of which came first after the domestication of barley—beer or bread?

There is other evidence that alcohol goes back at least to Paleolithic times. This derives from etymology as well as from studies of Stone Age cultures that survived into the twentieth century.

Presumably, fermented fruit juices (wine), fermented grains (beer), and fermented honey (mead) were available to Paleolithic man. Etymological evidence suggests that mead may have been the earliest beverage of choice. The word *mead* derives, by way of *mede* (Middle English) and *meodu* (Anglo-Saxon), from ancient words of Indo-European stock, such as *methyl* (Greek) and *madhu* (Sanskrit). In Sanskrit and Greek, the term means both 'honey' and 'intoxicating drink'. The association of honey, rather than grain or fruit, with intoxication may indicate its greater antiquity as a source of alcohol.

The majority of Stone Age cultures that survived into modern times have been familiar with alcohol. Early European explorers of Africa and the New World frequently discovered that alcohol was important in the local cultures. For instance, the Indians of eastern North America used alcohol in the form of fermented birch and sugar maple sap.

Alcohol has been used medicinally and in religious ceremonies for thousands of years, and it has a long history of recreational use. According to the Old Testament, Noah 'drank of the wine and was drunken'. Mesopotamian civilization provided one of the earliest clinical descriptions of intoxication and one of the first hangover cures.

Mesopotamian physicians advised as follows:

If a man has taken strong wine, his head is affected and he forgets his words and his speech becomes confused, his mind wanders and his eyes have a set of expression; to cure him, take licorice, beans, oleander ... to be compounded with oil and wine before the approach of the goddess Gula (or sunset), and in the morning before sunrise and before anyone has kissed him, let him take it, and he will recover.

One of the few surviving relics of the Seventeenth Egyptian Dynasty, which roughly coincided with the reign of Hammurabi, is a hieroglyphic outburst of a female courtier. 'Give me eighteen bowls of wine!' she exclaims for posterity. 'Behold, I love drunkenness!' So did other Egyptians of that era. Drunkenness was not rare, historians write, and seems to have occurred in all layers of society from the farmers to the gods (or ruling class). Banquets frequently ended with the guests, men and women, being sick, and this did not in any way seem shocking.

Not only are descriptions of drunkenness found in the historical record, but also pleas for moderation. Dynastic Egypt apparently invented the first temperance tract. Moderation was recommended by no less an authority on moderation than Genghis Khan: 'A soldier must not get drunk oftener than once a week. It would, of course, be better if he did not get drunk at all, but one should not expect the impossible'. The Old Testament condemns drunkenness, but not alcohol. 'Give strong drink unto him that is ready to perish', the Book of Proverbs proclaims, 'and wine unto those that be of heavy hearts. Let him drink, forget his poverty, and remember his misery no more'.

The 'strong drink' of the Bible was probably undiluted wine. 'She hath mingled her wine', reports Proverbs; a mixture of wine and water was the usual Jewish drink.

Alexander the Great was one of a long line of heavy-drinking generals. According to Plutarch, Alexander was under the influence of alcohol at the time of the burning of the royal palace at Persepolis in 330 BCE, seven years before his death. With torch in hand, a drunken Alexander led revelers in a procession in honor of Dionysus and threw the first firebrand, an act he bitterly regretted when sober. The final year of Alexander's life was punctuated with drunken binges, and his death may have been hastened by alcohol withdrawal.

Plutarch describes a mass orgy in 325 BCE involving Alexander and his Macedonian army: 'Not a single helmet, shield or spear was to be seen, but along the whole line of march the soldiers kept dipping their cups, drinking-horns or earthenware goblets into huge casks and mixing bowls and toasting one another, some drinking as they marched, others sprawled by the wayside'. The history of war is filled with similar scenes.

Alcohol has been the 'intoxicant of choice' in Judaeo-Christian culture. 'To drink is a Christian diversion/Unknown to the Turk and the Persian,' wrote Congreve 300 years ago. It was not *totally* unknown to the Turk and the Persian, but it is true that they favored other intoxicants, notably the products of the poppy and the hemp plant.

One of the myths of our times is that the 'stresses' of modern living have produced a society unusually reliant on alcohol. This is not true. Per capita consumption in the USA was highest, at an estimated six or seven gallons per person, in the early 1800s when whiskey was more portable than grain, and cider more portable than apples. Portability was important before trains came along, especially if you were westward bound in a covered wagon.

In the UK, drinking and drunkenness reached a peak during the 'gin epidemic' of the mid-eighteenth century, when gin sold for a few pennies a pint. Probably in no period of history have so many inebriates crowded the streets of a city as occurred in Hogarth's London. Less beer is consumed per capita in the UK now than 100 years ago. Consumption of wine *was* decreasing but started upward again in the late 1960s when the import fees were reduced and the influence of the European Common Market took hold.

Fluctuations in consumption have also been influenced by availability of potable water, the introduction of coffee, tea, and cocoa at prices the population could afford, and the waxing and waning of temperance movements.

Alcohol consumption has declined to some extent in recent years in the USA and most Western countries. There has been no change, apparently, in Russia and Poland. Today, in the USA, the reported consumption of alcohol (pure alcohol) is a little less than three gallons per person (over 14 years of age) per annum. This figure is based on tax data. Untaxed sales, such as those on military installations, are not included, and so per capita consumption may be under-estimated. Also, because consumption estimates are based on the resident population, when residents of one state cross into another state to purchase lower-priced alcoholic beverages, the result is a higher per capita consumption figure for the state in which sales occur. Washington DC and states with high rates of tourism and business travel have higher reported consumption rates because sales to transients are calculated as consumption by the resident population.

Any reductions in the consumption of alcohol in the USA have occurred despite the fact that people are drinking less untaxed alcohol. There is less available. Moonshine used to be a booming industry in some back country areas, especially during Prohibition, but no longer is today. Making moonshine alcohol was mainly a small family business, and small family businesses in the USA have declined. In more recent years, beer manufactured in local 'micro-breweries' has become popular.

There has been an interesting change in beverage preference. In diet-conscious America people drink more 'light' beer (beer with fewer calories) than regular beer. They also drink more 'white' spirits, such as vodka or gin, than 'brown' spirits (whiskey). The explanation for the latter is not clear, unless people have the notion that white spirits are healthier than brown, which is probably not true.

International comparisons are difficult at best. However, it appears that 'wine countries' such as France and Italy consume more alcohol than do countries where distilled spirits are favored. Israel has the lowest per capita consumption. Ireland, contrary to its popular image, has a lower consumption rate than the UK. The USA ranks in the middle with regard to alcohol consumption, and Russians are believed to be among the heaviest drinkers in the world despite 'official' government reports to the contrary.

Most adults in the USA are light drinkers. About 39 percent abstain, 42 percent drink less than three drinks per week, and only 5 percent consume an average of one ounce or more of alcohol per day.

Drinking patterns vary by age and sex. For both men and women, the prevalence of drinking is highest and abstention is lowest in the 18–24 year age range. Twice as many males are 'heavy' drinkers compared with females less than 65 years of age. For ages 65 years and older, abstainers equal drinkers in both genders and only 3 percent of men and women are considered heavy drinkers.

The level of consumption varies markedly in different segments of the population. Young white males drink more than any other group in the USA. The proportion of adolescents who report drinking increases steadily with age, with 75 percent of the oldest schoolchildren reporting some alcohol use. By that age 60 percent report being drunk at least once.

Consumption must be distinguished from alcoholism. Is the latter increasing? It is hard to say. There are several problems in estimating the prevalence of alcoholism. One is that few agree on the definition of alcoholism. Also, when a household survey is done, the alcoholics, more than most people, are not at home. Neighborhood bars are rarely included in household surveys.

Normal drinking

Throughout the ages (and throughout this book), a distinction has been made between normal and abnormal drinking. Before dealing at length with abnormal drinking (drinking that produces problems), something should be said about normal drinking.

How much can you drink and still be 'normal'?

Normal can be defined in several ways. It can be defined as drinking no more than 'society' deems safe and prudent, i.e. normal. Since societies vary in this regard, the definition is not very helpful.

According to another definition, normal drinking is drinking less than is required to produce medical, social, or psychological problems. The problem definition also has problems, as will be discussed later.

Finally, attempts are made from time to time to separate normal from abnormal drinking in terms of quantity of alcohol consumed. A nineteenth-century British physician named Dr Anstie proclaimed that normal drinking consisted of drinking no more than three ounces of whiskey or half a bottle of table wine or two pints of beer a day (known for years as 'Dr Anstie's limits').

In 1990 the US Government defined normal drinking somewhat more conservatively. It defined moderate drinking (a synonym for normal) as no more than one drink a day for most women and no more than two drinks a day for most men. A 'drink' was defined as 12 ounces of beer, 5 ounces of wine, or 1.5 ounces of 80-proof distilled spirits. Each of these drinks contain about the same amount of absolute alcohol—1 ounce or 12 grams.

The government points out that even this amount of alcohol should be avoided by some people. These include women who are pregnant or trying to conceive, people who drive or engage in activities that require attention or skill, people taking medications, including over-the-counter medications, recovering alcoholics, and persons under the age of 21.

As noted, women become more intoxicated than men on an equivalent dose of alcohol. This is apparently due to a difference in the activity of an enzyme in the stomach that breaks down alcohol before it reaches the bloodstream. The enzyme is four times more active in men than in women. Women also have proportionally more fat and less body water than men. Because alcohol is more soluble in water than in fat, a particular dose of alcohol becomes more highly concentrated in a female's body than in a male's. This may explain why female alcoholics tend to suffer more damaging health effects with less overall alcohol exposure than do men.

Authorities concede that a small amount of alcohol may be beneficial. Alcohol reduces tension, anxiety, and self-consciousness. It promotes conviviality. In the elderly, moderate drinking stimulates appetite, promotes regular bowel function, and improves mood. In addition, there is considerable evidence that moderate drinking decreases the risk of death from coronary artery disease. In one study, American men who drank three drinks per day were less likely to die than men who reported abstinence; they had fewer heart attacks. In another study, one drink a day decreased the risk of coronary heart disease in middle-aged women. These benefits appear to be the result of favorable effects of alcohol consumption on blood lipid profiles. Moderate drinking increases the levels of high-density lipoproteins (HDLs), the so called 'good' cholesterol, in the blood and decreases the levels of total cholesterol and low-density lipoprotein (LDL) cholesterol, the so-called 'bad' cholesterol.[1] Moderate drinking also reduces the body's ability to form blood clots.

The beneficial effects of drinking are achieved at fairly low levels of alcohol consumption. Even moderate drinking has risks that might offset these benefits. Low levels of alcohol consumption have been reported to increase blood pressure and the risk of strokes caused by bleeding (hemorrhagic strokes). This is at odds with the statement that alcohol in moderate amounts decreases the risk of strokes caused by blocked blood vessels (ischemic strokes). Impairment of driving skills by alcohol may begin at low blood alcohol concentrations, especially when the drinker is fatigued or taking drugs. Among drugs that strengthen alcohol's effects are sleeping pills, tranquilizers, anticonvulsants, antidepressants, and some painkillers. Small amounts of alcohol may help prevent coronary disease, but in severe heart failure alcohol may only worsen the condition and interfere with the function of medications that are used to treat the disease.

Heavy drinking is associated with an increased risk of certain types of cancer, mostly cancers of the liver and digestive system. One study indicated that breast cancer was twice as likely to develop in women who drank three to nine drinks per week than in women who drank fewer than three drinks per week. In many cases, the increased risk of cancer can be offset completely by supplementation with a specific vitamin, folic acid. This suggests that the natural 'cause' of alcohol-related cancers may be the poor nutritional status of most alcoholics and not directly due to alcohol consumption. Malnutrition is a particular problem for the alcoholic, contributing to a number of alcoholism-related maladies. Nutritional factors that are relevant to alcoholism were discussed in Chapter 2. Most researchers still believe that the inflammatory effects of excessive alcohol consumption contribute to the development of cancers. Alcohol also promotes the growth of blood vessels within tumors, which may fuel the growth of a cancer once it forms.

Adverse effects of alcohol on the fetus have been reported. These effects are usually, but not always, associated with heavy consumption of alcohol during pregnancy. One study found that consumption of two or three drinks per day during pregnancy was associated with low birth-weight and minor physical anomalies. Women who drank alcohol during their pregnancy were also more likely to experience an extremely premature birth (prior to 26 weeks) which in itself places the infant at risk for a host of developmental problems. Another study reported that women drinking two drinks per day during pregnancy had children with lower IQs. Animal research provides additional evidence for adverse fetal effects at low levels of drinking. This research has resulted in the warning label placed on all alcoholic beverages that cautions women to avoid drinking alcohol during pregnancy. The fetal alcohol syndrome will be discussed further in Chapter 8.

Unfortunately, moderate drinking does not always remain moderate. Some moderate drinkers progress to heavy drinking and some become alcoholic, as defined in the next chapter. This book is mainly about alcoholism. Even so, it is important to remember that alcohol-related problems can occur in people who are not alcoholic. For some people, there is no such thing as moderate drinking.

Section 2

Alcoholism

In my judgment such of us who have never fallen victims [to alcoholism] have been spared more by the absence of appetite than from any mental or moral superiority over those who have. Indeed, I believe if we take habitual drunkards as a class, their heads and the hearts will bear an advantageous comparison with those of any class.

Abraham Lincoln

He drank, not as an epicure, but barbarously, with a speed and dispatch altogether American, as if he were performing homicidal function, as if he had to kill something inside himself, a worm that would not die.

Baudelaire, writing about Edgar Allan Poe

5

What is alcoholism?

An alcoholic is a person who drinks, has problems from drinking, but goes on drinking anyway.

 Patient's perspective

I am David. I am an alcoholic. I have always been an alcoholic. I will always be an alcoholic. I cannot touch alcohol. It will destroy me. It is like an allergy—not a real allergy—but like an allergy.

I had my first drink at 16. I got drunk. For several years I drank every week or so with the boys. I didn't always get drunk, but I know now that alcohol affected me differently than other people. I looked forward to the times I knew I could drink. I drank for the glow, the feeling of confidence it gave me. But maybe that's why my friends drank too. They didn't become alcoholics. Alcohol seemed to satisfy some specific need I had, which I can't describe. True, it made me feel good, helped me forget my troubles, but that wasn't it. What was it? I don't know, but I know I liked it, and after a time, I more than liked it, I needed it. Of course, I didn't realize it. It was maybe 10 or 15 years before I realized it, let myself realize it.

My need was easy to hide from myself and others (maybe I'm kidding myself about the others). I only associated with people who drank. I married a woman who drank. There were always reasons to drink. I was low, tense, tired, mad, happy. I probably drank as often because I was happy as for any other reason. And occasions for drinking—when drinking was appropriate, expected—were endless. Football games, fishing trips, parties, holidays, birthdays, Christmas, or merely Saturday night. Drinking became interwoven with everything pleasurable—food, sex, social life. When I stopped drinking, these things, for a time, lost all interest for me, they were so tied to drinking. I don't think I will ever enjoy them as much as I did when drinking. But if I had kept drinking, I wouldn't be here to enjoy them. I would be dead.

So, drinking came to dominate my life. By the time I was 25, I was drinking every day, usually before dinner, but sometimes after dinner (if there was a 'reason'), and more on weekends, starting in the afternoon. By 30, I drank all weekend, starting with a beer or Bloody Mary in the morning, and drinking off and on, throughout the day, beer or wine or vodka indiscriminately. The goal, always, was to maintain a glow, not enough, I hoped, that people would notice, but a glow. When 5 o'clock came, I thought, well, now it's cocktail hour and I would have my two or three scotches or martinis before dinner as I did on non-weekend nights. After dinner I might nap, but just as often felt a kind of wakeful calm and power and happiness that I've never experienced any other time. These were the dangerous moments. I called friends, boring them with drunken talk; arranged parties; decided impulsively to drive to a bar. In one year, at the age of 33, I had three accidents, all on Saturday night, and was charged with drunken driving once (I kept my license, but barely). My friends became fewer, reduced to other heavy drinkers and barflies. I fought with my wife, blaming her for her drinking, and once or twice hit her (or so she said—like many things I did while drinking, there was no memory afterward).

And by now I was drinking at noontime, with the lunch hour stretching longer and longer. I began taking off whole afternoons, going home potted. I missed mornings at work because of drinking the night before, particularly Monday mornings. And I began drinking weekday mornings to get going. Vodka and orange juice. I thought vodka wouldn't smell (it did). It usually lasted until an early martini luncheon, and I then suffered through until cocktail hour, which came earlier and earlier.

By now I was hooked and knew it, but desperately did not want others to know it. I had been sneaking drinks for years—slipping out to the kitchen during parties and such—but now I began hiding alcohol, in my desk, bedroom, car glove compartment, so it would never be far away, ever. I grew panicky even thinking I might not have alcohol when I needed it, which was just about always.

For years, I drank and had very little hangover, but now the hangovers were gruesome. I felt physically bad—headachy, nauseous, weak—but the mental part was the hardest. I loathed myself. I was waking early and thinking what a mess I was, how I had hurt so many others and myself. The word 'guilty' and 'depression' sound superficial in trying to describe how I felt. The loathing was almost physical—a dead weight that could be lifted in only one way, and that was by having a drink, so I drank, morning after morning. After two or three, my hands were steady, I could hold some breakfast down, and the guilt was gone, or almost.

Despite everything, others knew. There was the odor, the rheumy eyes, and flushed face. There was missing work and not working well when there. Fights with my wife, increasingly physical. She kept threatening to leave and finally did. My boss gave me a leave of absence after an embarrassed remark about my 'personal problems'. At some point I was without wife, home, or job. I had nothing to do but drink. The drinking was now steady, days on end. I lost appetite and missed meals (besides, money was short). I awoke at night, sweating and shaking, and had a drink. I awoke in the morning vomiting and had a drink. It couldn't last. My ex-wife found me in my apartment shaking and seeing things, and got me in the hospital. I dried out, left, and went back to drinking. I was hospitalized again, and this time stayed dry for 6 months. I was nervous and couldn't sleep, but got some of my confidence back and found a part-time job. Then my ex-boss offered my job back and I celebrated by having a drink. The next night I had two drinks. In a month I was drinking as much as ever and again unemployed. That was 3 years ago. I've had two big drinks since then but don't drink other times. I think about alcohol and miss it. Life is gray and monotonous. The joy and gaiety are gone. But drinking will kill me. I know this and have stopped—for now.

A tree is known by its fruit; alcoholism by its problems. Theoretically, a person can drink a gallon of whiskey a day for a lifetime, not have problems, and therefore not be alcoholic. Theoretically. In fact, heavy drinkers almost always have problems. Sometimes they are mild. Alcohol calories may result in excess weight—a cosmetic if not a medical problem. Things may be said while drinking that would not or should not be said at other times. A minor traffic offence may have major consequences when alcohol is on the breath.

Problems yes, but alcoholism? The verdict rests with the observer. A fundamentalist teetotaler may view any problem from drinking as alcoholism. Moderate drinkers may be more indulgent, saying in effect: 'These things happen. If they do not happen too often, it probably does not mean much'. But what is too often? Except in extreme cases (the Davids, about whom everyone agrees) there will always be controversy about who is and who is not an alcoholic. This is understandable; doctors disagree about who has heart disease if the case is mild.

'Alcoholism' in this book refers to the David type of alcoholism, granting that patterns of human behavior are bewilderingly variable, even patterns of illness. Not all Davids, for example, reach bottom. Some stop drinking long before. Others drink, but with enough control to prevent the big problems from happening. The essence of the David type of alcoholism is a vulnerability to alcohol that sets him apart from other drinkers. By taking extreme measures, such as total abstinence, he may prevent alcohol problems; but if he drinks at all, the chance of developing problems is high, and this vulnerability appears to be lifelong.

How many people have this condition? It depends. Population surveys show that about 62 percent of adults in the USA drink. About 7 percent (11 percent of men, 3 percent of women) drink 'heavily', meaning that they drink almost daily and enough to be somewhat intoxicated several times a month. About 9 percent have problems from drinking, mostly minor; another 9 percent have had problems in the past. (There seems to be considerable migration in and out of the 'problem-drinking' pool.) Among the problem drinkers are a subgroup called alcoholics. How many alcoholics are there? Nobody knows, but undoubtedly alcoholics like David exist in large numbers in all Western countries.

These figures have remained fairly consistent in the USA over the past 20 years, with, as noted, an overall decline in consumption, at least by non-alcoholic drinkers. It is interesting to compare the situation in the USA with that in the UK. In the late 1980s the World Health Organization sponsored a survey of nine countries, inquiring about drinking problems. The results appeared in a report by the Institute of Medicine in the USA called *Broadening the base of treatment for alcohol problems*. (National Academy Press, Washington DC, 1990). The report from the UK came from R. Hodgson of Cardiff. Marcus Grant and E.B. Ritson, both of the World Health Organization, were responsible for preparing the summary.

Based on government data, it was estimated that about 10 percent of adults in the UK were heavy drinkers. Thirty adults per 1000 admitted to having problems from drinking. Five adults per 1000 were problem drinkers. One adult per 2000 was admitted to a psychiatric hospital with an alcohol-related diagnosis. Most of the problem drinkers were male. However, medical complications of drinking were increasing faster among women than among men. In the 1980s, deaths from liver disease rose by 9 percent in women compared with a 1 percent fall for men. There was also a large increase in the number of women seeking alcohol counseling services. The 18–24 age group had the highest proportion of heavy drinkers. There was a marked rise in teenage drunkenness. Recent data have indicated a gradual rise in the consumption of alcohol in the UK, particularly among young drinkers (boys and girls), since the early 1990s.

Alcohol consumption in most Westernized countries appears to be declining. However, drinking in poor and developing countries has risen steadily since the early 1970s. Again, nobody knows how many alcoholics like David exist in the UK or the world. The true number is ultimately dictated by the definition of the problem, which clearly varies.

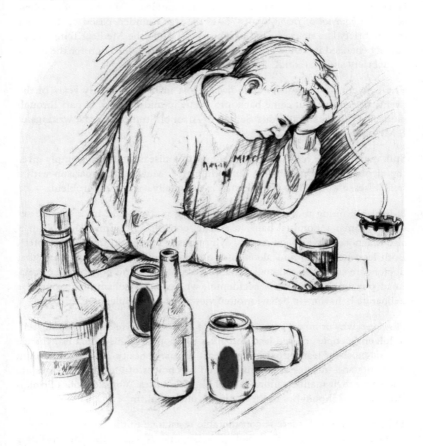

Figure 1.1 'Troubled drinker'. Artwork by Lorie Gavulic.

A disease?

Is alcoholism a disease? The question arises frequently and is the subject of fierce debate among alcoholism experts.

A little historical background may help to put the matter in perspective. The 'disease concept' of alcoholism is not new. It originated in the writings of Benjamin Rush and the British physician Thomas Trotter in the early nineteenth century and became increasingly popular with physicians as the century progressed. In the 1930s, Dr Samuel Woodward, the first superintendent of Worcester State Hospital, Massachusetts, and Dr Eli Tood of Hartford, Connecticut, established the first medical institutions for inebriates. The *Journal of Inebriety* (1876–1914) was founded based on the 'fact that inebriety is a neurosis and psychosis'. In 1904 the Medical Temperance Society changed its name to the American Medical Association for the Study of Inebriety and Narcotics.

The concept of alcoholism as a disease lost favor in the early years of the twentieth century, but came back into vogue in mid-century, in part through pioneering studies at the Yale School of Alcohol Studies and the writings of E.M. Jellinek.

Still, many people resist. Calling alcoholism a disease, they say, simply gives the alcoholic a good alibi for self-indulgence. Maybe a comparison with a 'real' disease would help resolve what is essentially a semantic problem.

Is lead poisoning a disease? Lead poisoning is diagnosed by a specific set of symptoms: abdominal pain, headache, convulsions, coma. Alcoholism is also diagnosed by a specific set of symptoms (reviewed in the next chapter). Both lead poisoning and alcoholism are 'medical' problems, meaning that doctors are supposed to know something about them and possibly be of help. Lead poisoning is typically accidental, whereas alcoholism arises out of a deliberate behavior—a behavior often viewed as self-indulgent, even sinful.

However, why or how a person 'catches' a disease is not relevant. If some 'self-indulgent' people enjoyed lead and ate it like popcorn, this would not change the diagnosis of lead intoxication. Heart disease, obesity, diabetes, and even accidents and injuries are all influenced by choices of lifestyle. Diseases are known by their manifestations as well as their causes. Why alcoholics drink is irrelevant (or should be) to the diagnosis of alcoholism.

Still, as mentioned, there is considerable resistance to the disease concept—particularly on the part of psychologists. Opponents believe that 'medicalizing' what is essentially an aberrant form of behaviors—or bad set of habits—is wrong. They point out that millions of people have bad effects from drinking and are not alcoholic by anyone's definition. Nevertheless, they deserve understanding, study, and sometimes professional help. These people, for the purposes of this book, will be called *problem drinkers*, or persons with alcohol-related problems who do not meet the criteria for alcoholism. Some of these problems may be medical, social, or psychiatric, but they are caused or worsened by alcohol and the person continues to drink *despite* this.

Thus, even with the problem drinker (the person who becomes socially gauche on one drink or suffers excruciating heartburn), the fact that he or she drinks anyway suggests that there is an element of compulsion in the drinking—just as there is in the most severe form of problem drinking still called, by many, alcoholism (or sometimes alcohol dependence).

Alcoholism is a compulsion to drink that leads to a breakdown in the victim's ability to function. He suffers more than heartburn or social embarrassment. Alcohol, for the alcoholic, is a lethal poison, a destroyer of the person's ability to lead anything resembling a normal existence. Alcohol, for the alcoholic, becomes an overpowering obsession that leads to a compulsion to drink that is so strong that it dominates his life. Obtaining the next drink becomes a need that obliterates every other aspect of a person's psychological being and the alcoholic's body comes to depend on alcohol almost as much as it depends on oxygen and food.

This is the working definition of alcoholism used in this book. According to this definition, David was an alcoholic.

The critics of the disease concept are right in one regard. Some people have a drinking problem who are not alcoholic by the above definition, and never will be. The non-alcoholic problem drinker is also the subject of this book.

6

The symptoms

> **Key points**
>
> - The disease of alcoholism can be characterized by series of specific psychological, medical, and social symptoms.
>
> - The psychological symptoms of alcoholism are defined by an increasing obsession with finding and consuming alcohol.
>
> - Alcoholic drinking triggers a cascade of biochemical changes in the body which can lead to the development of a variety of medical syndromes, the combination of which may differ from person to person.
>
> - The broad effects of alcoholism on the individual, their family, and society at large amount to a tremendous social and economic burden.

This chapter is mainly about alcoholics, heavy drinkers for whom drinking has become a central activity in their way of life. However, many non-alcoholics have experienced some of the problems addressed below, and these will be discussed at the end of the chapter.

Psychological problems

The symptoms of alcoholism fall into three groups: psychological, medical, and social. We shall start with those that are psychological.

Preoccupation with alcohol

The alcoholic thinks about alcohol from morning till night, and at night, if not too drunk to dream, dreams about alcohol. When to have the first drink?

When the next? Remember the times that bars will be closed. Prepare, prepare. Will they sell more than two drinks on the plane? Take a flask. Do the Smiths drink? Find out before accepting their dinner invitation. This goes on and on, blotting out other thoughts, other plans.

It is obsessional in precisely the way that psychiatrists use the word. Obsessions breed compulsions, and when an alcoholic drops into a bar or nightclub, ever so casually, it is as compulsive as the neurotic washing his hands for the twentieth time that day.

Self-deception

But he must not admit it to himself. 'We are all victims of systematic self-deception', Santayana said, and the alcoholic is a victim *par excellence*. People are victims of many things—cancer, lust, society—and can accept it. But, deep down, the alcoholic believes he is doing it to himself; he is the perpetrator, not the victim. And this he cannot accept, so he lies to himself.

'I can stop drinking any time. Important people drink. Churchill drank. Today is special—a friend is in town. Nothing is going on—why not? Life is tragic—why not? Tomorrow we die—why not?'

As he lies to himself, he lies to others, and concealment becomes a game like the one children play when they raid the cookie jar and hope their mother won't notice.

Guilt

But he does know and can't help knowing. There are too many reminders. The wife's pleas and tantrums. The boss's 'friendly' advice. The dented bumper. The night terrors and night sweats. The trembling hands. The puffy eyes and blotchy complexion. The terrifying memory gaps. All spell self-destruction, and even the cleverest self-deceiver knows it.

Amnesia

Alcoholics have memory lapses when they drink, and this is often attributed to guilt. It is said that the forgetter does not want to remember. Non-alcoholics also have memory lapses when they drink, not so often or so severely, but non-alcoholics by definition drink less. Memory lapses (or blackouts, as they are called when alcohol is involved) are probably not due to guilt. More likely alcohol, in some people on some occasions, interferes with chemical processes that make memory (perhaps the most mysterious of biological phenomena) possible.

Precisely how it occurs is unknown, but the memory lapses are genuine. The drinker does things when he is drinking that ordinarily he would remember perfectly, but when he sobers up, usually the next day, he has no recollection of what he has done. Sometimes he realizes that he had a memory lapse. He is apprehensive. He checks to see if his car is in the garage. He looks for dents that weren't there before. His over-riding fear is that he did something—broke a law, harmed someone—and punishment is at hand. He retraces his movements of the night before. 'Was I here, Joe?' he asks. Told that he was: 'What did I do? Was I drunk?' Reassured that he did nothing wrong and was no more drunk than usual, he goes to the next place where he might have been. Alternatively, he may avoid all places and all companions he might have visited or been with during the forgotten interval, preferring not to know.

In truth, people rarely do things during blackouts that they don't also do when they are drunk and suffer no memory loss.

During blackouts, the person is conscious and alert. He may appear normal. He may do complicated things—converse intelligently, seduce strangers, travel.

Case study

A 39-year-old salesman awoke in a strange hotel room. He had a mild hangover but otherwise felt normal. His clothes were hanging in the closet; he was clean-shaven. He dressed and went down to the lobby. He learned from the clerk that he was in Las Vegas and that he had checked in two days previously. It had been obvious that he had been drinking, the clerk said, but he hadn't seemed very drunk. The date was Saturday the 14th. His last recollection was of sitting in a St Louis bar on Monday the 9th. He had been drinking all day and was drunk, but could remember everything perfectly until about 3 p.m. when, 'like a curtain dropping', his memory went blank. It remained blank for approximately five days. Three years later, it was still blank. He was so frightened by the experience that he abstained from alcohol for two years.

Some people forget and do not realize when sober that they have forgotten anything. Someone tells them and then they remember a little.

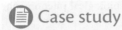 Case study

A 53-year-old member of Alcoholics Anonymous said that he had experienced many blackouts during his 25 years of heavy drinking. He could not remember his first blackout, but guessed it had happened about 15 years before. The memory loss had not bothered him, he said; he assumed that everyone who drank had trouble with memory. Sometimes, however, it was embarrassing to be told he had said something or gone somewhere and not recalled it. Upon being told, he would sometimes remember the event and sometimes not. Occasionally, months later, something would remind him of the event and his memory would 'snap back'. Typically, he could remember some parts of a drinking episode and not others; a half hour might be blanked out and the next hour remembered. The forgotten parts appeared to have no more emotional significance than the remembered ones. 'It's like turning a switch on and off.'

Sometimes a curious thing happens when a person is drinking: the drinker recalls things that happened during a previous drinking period which, when sober, he had forgotten. For example, alcoholics often report hiding money or alcohol when drinking, forgetting it when sober, and having their memory return when drinking again. This phenomenon is referred to as 'state-dependent learning'. Whatever the explanation, the mind does play odd tricks on drinkers:

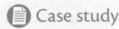 Case study

A 47-year-old housewife often wrote letters when she was drinking. Sometimes she would jot down notes for a letter and start writing it but not finish it. The next day, sober, she would be unable to decipher the notes. Then she would start drinking again, and after a few drinks the meaning of the notes would become clear and she would resume writing the letter. 'It was like picking up the pencil where I had left off.'

Anxiety and depression

What goes up comes down, and alcoholic euphoria is followed by alcoholic depression with a kind of Newtonian inevitability. Anxiety and depression occur not only with hangovers but intermittently during the drinking period itself, if the drinking is heavy and continuous. This sequence is common: a man feels bad for any reason (it's a gray day); he drinks, and feels better;

then he feels bad again, this time because the alcohol effect is wearing off; he drinks again, feels better again. A vicious circle is under way, based on alcohol's ability to raise and lower spirits alternately. This roller-coaster effect is probably chemical in nature, but the drinker only knows that alcohol, having raised his spirits, now lowers them, and that the best way to raise them again is to have another drink.

Medical problems

If this process goes on long enough, there are usually medical problems. They may take years to develop, and some lucky drinkers are never affected. Incredibly, a person may consume a ferocious quantity of alcohol, maybe a fifth or quart of whiskey a day for 20 years or longer, and when he dies a 'natural' death, his brain, liver, pancreas, and coronary arteries appear normal. But the odds are strong that something will give. Here are some favorite targets.

The stomach

Gastritis, inflammation of the stomach's lining, is common. The symptoms are gas, bloating, heartburn, and nausea. Alcohol's role in producing stomach or duodenal ulcers has become clearer in recent years.

Ulcers are caused by hydrochloric acid and digestive enzymes. These are powerful enough to digest fish bones and the toughest beefsteak, but do not digest the stomach itself. The mucous lining of the stomach somehow prevents it. When the protection is lost, ulcers develop. This can sometimes occur as a result of a bacterial infection.[1] If alcohol, hot peppers, or pent-up anger produce ulcers at all, they must do so by either increasing acid production or breaching the protective barrier. Alcohol, in concentrated doses, decreases rather than increases acid production. Stronger alcohol solutions (over 10 percent alcohol) appear to damage the gastric mucosa directly. The selection of drink may be important in this regard because, in controlled tests, alcoholic beverages did less damage than mixtures of pure ethyl alcohol. It may be that some of the congeners in alcoholic beverages, especially beer and wine, offer the stomach lining some measure of protection from the corrosive effects of straight alcohol.

The liver

The word 'cirrhosis' comes from the Greek word for yellow-orange, probably because people with cirrhosis become jaundiced. Alcoholics are disposed to a type of cirrhosis called portal cirrhosis, or Laennec's cirrhosis.

In the first stages of cirrhosis, liver cells become inflamed and gradually die out. The liver swells up and can be felt through the belly wall, whereas usually it is hidden behind the ribs. New cells appear (the body is incorrigibly bent on keeping things going), but with a difference. Previously the cells lined up in columns, forming banks for concentric canals through which blood coursed. The new cells form higgledy-piggledy, and the blood flow almost comes to a halt.

The results are predictable. Blood backs up and seeps into the abdomen, which swells like a balloon, or it detours around the liver, engorging the paper-thin veins of the esophagus. If the veins burst, fatal hemorrhage may result. The liver cells, formerly little factories with many functions, go on strike and their production of proteins, blood-clotting factors, and other vital constituents falls off. In men, the cells no longer suppress female sex hormones (even the manliest of men has *some* female hormones), and so men's breasts grow, their testicles shrink, and they lose their baritone voices, beards, and hairy chests. As the process continues, scar tissue forms and eventually the liver is like a small lumpy rock, incapable of sustaining life.

Alcoholic cirrhosis, formerly called Laennec's cirrhosis, is the most common type of cirrhosis. However, most alcoholics do not develop cirrhosis, and the connection between drinking and cirrhosis is still not understood.

The risk of liver disease increases when certain drugs are taken together. Carbon tetrachloride and other halogenated hydrocarbons can produce liver damage alone, but when they are combined with alcohol the risk of liver damage is much greater. Acute and sometimes catastrophic liver disease has occurred in individuals who devote a Saturday afternoon to scrubbing their wall-to-wall carpets with a cleaning fluid while drinking half a case of beer.

Nerve fibers

The long nerve fibers extending from the spinal cord to muscles often suffer degenerative changes in alcoholics. These changes interrupt the smooth communication between nerve fibers. The fibers make muscles contract and maintain muscular tone; they also transmit back to the spinal cord, and thence the brain, messages from sensory receptors in muscle and skin. The degeneration of nerves results in muscular weakness and eventual wasting and paralysis. Pain and tingling are experienced, and there may be eventual loss of sensation. As discussed in Chapter 2, the cause of nerve fiber degeneration in the alcoholic is not alcohol; it is a vitamin deficiency. High doses of B vitamins may restore the fibers to their normal state, if not given too late.

Brain damage

After many years of heavy drinking, most alcoholics, when recovered from their latest drinking bout, show little or no sign of intellectual impairment. Their IQs are normal, their thoughts logical, and their minds clear. If there is impairment, it is usually subtle, rarely persists, and can be attributed to factors other than loss of brain cells—poor motivation, for example, in taking the tests that psychologists are forever giving alcoholics.

Imaging techniques, including computed X-rays of the brain (CAT scans) and magnetic resonance imaging (MRI), have been applied to alcoholics in several studies. The results are mixed. Most do report some degree of shrinkage of brain tissue in response to alcohol exposure. These effects appear to increase with age and alcohol consumption. The loss can be reversed to some degree with abstinence, but recovery rarely returns the alcoholic's brain size to that of non-alcoholics (although the young do appear to bounce back somewhat better).

However, these differences in brain size do not necessarily predict mental ability, because alcoholics and non-alcoholics appear to lose their mental capabilities at the same rate as they age. It is interesting to note that alcoholics may have smaller brains than non-alcoholics even before they start drinking. Some differences have been observed in measures of brain growth which may be related to inherited factors that influence the risk of becoming alcoholic in the first place. These differences in brain size have also been correlated with decreases in some measures of mental ability in alcoholics. The true relationship between brain size and intellect is still controversial. After all, the brains of women are generally smaller than the brains of men, and this is not considered to reflect a difference in mental ability.

A small minority of alcoholics definitely suffer brain damage due to deficiency of thiamine, a B vitamin. The malnourished alcoholic gets too little thiamine, and if the deprivation persists and is severe, certain well-demarcated areas of the brain are destroyed. These areas are definitely involved in memory storage. Their destruction results in severe memory impairment. A German named Wernicke and a Russian named Korsakoff first described the disease. The patient with Wernicke–Korsakoff disease can remember the distant past fairly well, has a normal IQ, and seems reasonably bright; however, he is unable to remember anything that happened to him a few minutes after it happens. The condition is devastating, and the chronic Wericke–Korsakoff patient needs custodial care for the rest of his life. Thiamine, given early, may prevent a permanent defect. Fortunately, the condition is rare.

Alcoholics are also inclined to suffer degenerative nerve changes in the cerebellum, the half-melon bulge at the base of the brain that regulates coordination. An unsteady gait results. Thiamine deficiency is also believed to be the cause.

Impotence

> Macduff: What three things does drink especially provoke?
>
> Porter: Marry, sir, nose-painting, sleep and urine. Lechery, sir, it provokes, and unprovokes; it provokes the desire, but it takes away the performance ...
>
> *Macbeth* (Act II, scene iii)

Shakespeare names not three but four of alcohol's well-known actions, lechery being the most famous. By dilating blood vessels, alcohol 'paints' the nose; it makes people sleepy; and one of the things a novice drinker first notices about drink, it increases the need to urinate.

It also increases sexual desire. More accurately, perhaps, it 'releases' sexual desire—the well-known disinhibiting effect of alcohol. But performance may be impaired. Drunken men have trouble achieving an erection or ejaculation. Whether sexual performance in drunken women is also impaired is harder to determine. Some alcoholics not only have trouble with sexual performance when drinking, but the problem persists long into sobriety

As discussed in Chapter 2, alcohol suppresses testosterone production in men and estrogen release in women. Continued drinking, especially in adolescence, can irreversibly alter hormone regulation, resulting in changes in sexual performance, sexual characteristics, and fertility.

The alcohol-withdrawal syndrome

Alcoholics experience a medical problem which, strictly speaking, does not come from drinking alcohol but from not drinking alcohol. This is the alcohol-withdrawal syndrome. It is commonly, but mistakenly, called the DTs, or delirium tremens. In medical usage, 'delirium' means gross memory disturbance, usually combined with insomnia, agitation, hallucinations, and illusions. Most alcoholics do not experience delirium.

As a rule, alcohol withdrawal is a distressing but temporary condition lasting from two days to a week. The mildest symptom is shakiness, which begins a few hours after the alcoholic stops drinking, sometimes awakening him during sleep. Morning shakes are inevitable if the drinker has been drinking enough. His eyelids flutter and his tongue quivers, but most conspicuously his hands shake, so that transporting a cup of coffee from saucer to mouth is a major undertaking. The cure for the shakes, as for all alcohol-withdrawal symptoms, is a drink or two.

After a day or two without drinking, the alcoholic coming off a bender may start hallucinating—seeing and hearing things that others do not see or hear. He often realizes that he is hallucinating and blames alcohol. Not always, however. Sometimes the hallucinations are vivid, frightening, and as real as life.

Occasionally alcoholics have convulsions resembling the grand mal seizures of the epileptic. Most alcoholics are not epileptic and have seizures only when withdrawing from alcohol. The seizures usually occur one to three days after the person stops drinking.

The most severe form of withdrawal involves delirium and justifies using the term delirium tremens, the 'tremens' referring to the shakiness. Delirium is ominous. It often means the person not only has withdrawal symptoms but also a serious medical illness, often of the type to which alcoholics, because of their way of living, are vulnerable: pneumonia, fractures, blood clots in the brain, liver failure. People occasionally die in delirium tremens, whereas death from milder forms of withdrawal is rare.

Many alcoholics are capable of withdrawing from alcohol on their own. They often do this by tapering off—gradually decreasing the amount they drink. However, serious withdrawal symptoms justify hospitalization so that the alcoholic can be given tranquilizers to make him feel better, vitamins to prevent brain damage, and frequent medical examinations to exclude medical illness.

The DTs have been described brilliantly in fiction by, among others, Malcolm Lowry and Mark Twain. Lowry, in his novella *Lunar caustic*,[2] wrote from personal experience how it felt to wake up in an alcoholic ward.

The man awoke certain that he was on a ship. If not, where did those isolated clangings come from, those sounds of iron on iron? He recognized the crunch of water pouring over the scuttle, the heavy tramp of feet on the deck above, the steady Frére *Jacques*: Frére *Jacques* of the engines. He was on a ship, taking him back to England, which he never should have left in the first place. Now he was conscious of this racked, trembling, malodorous body. Daylight sent probes of agony against his eyelids. Opening them, he saw three negro sailors vigorously washing down the deck. He shut his eyes again. Impossible, he thought ...

As day grew, the noise became more ghastly: what sounded like a railway seemed to be running just over the ceiling. Another night came. The noise grew worse and, stranger yet, the crew kept multiplying. More and more men, bruised, wounded, and always drunk, were hurled down the alley by petty officers to lie his face downward, screaming or suddenly asleep on their hard bunks.

He was awake. What had he done last night? Nothing at all, perhaps, yet remorse tore at his vitals. He needed a drink desperately. He did not know whether his eyes were closed or open. Horrid shapes plunged out of the blankness, gibbering, rubbing their bristles against his face, but he couldn't move. Something had got under his bed too, a bear that kept trying to get up. Voices, a prosopopoeia of voices, murmured in his ears, ebbed away, murmured again, cackled, shrieked, cajoled; voices pleading with him to stop drinking, to die and be damned. Thronged, dreadful shadows came close, were snatched away. A cataract of water was pouring through the wall, filling the room. A red hand gesticulated, prodded him: over a ravaged mountain side of swift stream was carrying with it legless bodies yelling out of great eye-sockets, in which were broken teeth. Music mounted to screech, subsided. On a tumbled bloodstained bed in a house whose face was blasted away a large scorpion was gravely raping a one-armed negress. His wife appeared, tears streaming down her face, pitying, only to be instantly transformed into Richard III, who sprang forward to smother him.

After a few days, the DTs go away. Lowry's patient:

now knew himself to be in a kind of hospital, and with this realization everything became coherent and fell into place. The sound of water pouring over the scuttle was the terrific shock of the flushing toilet; the banging of iron and the dispersed noises, the rattling of keys, explained themselves; the frantic ringing of bells was for doctors or nurses; and all the shouting, shuffling, creaking and ordering was no more than the complex routine of the institution.

Lunar caustic

Psychiatric patients are rarely dangerous, but delirious patients are an exception. They may be dangerous indeed, as was the case of Huckleberry Finn's alcoholic father, whose DTs were described by Mark Twain as follows.

I don't know how long I was asleep, but all of a sudden there was an awful scream and I was up. There was Pap looking wild, and skipping around and yelling about snakes. I couldn't see no snakes, but he said they was crawling up his legs; and then he could give a jump and scream, and say one had bit him on the cheek. I never see a man look so wild. Pretty soon he was all fagged out, and fell down panting; then he rolled over and over, screaming and saying there was devils a-hold of him. He wore out by and by, and laid still awhile, moaning. Then he laid stiller, and didn't make a sound. I could hear the owls and the wolves away off in the woods, and it seemed terrible still. He was laying over by the corner. By and by, he raised up partway and listened, with his head to one side. He wails, very low:

'Tramp-tramp-tramp; that's the dead; tramp-tramp-tramp, they're coming after me; but I won't go. Oh, they're here! Don't touch me—don't. Hands off—they're cold; let go. Oh, let a poor devil alone!'

He rolled himself up on his blanket and went to crying. But by and by he rolled out and jumped up to his feet looking wild, and he see me and went for me. He chased me round and round the place with a clasp knife, calling me the Angel of Death, and saying he would kill me ... I begged, him, and told him I was only Huck; but he laughed such a screech laugh, and roared and cussed, and kept on chasing me. Once when I turned short and dodged under his arm he got me by the jacket between my shoulders, and I thought I was gone; but I slid out of the jacket and saved myself. Pretty soon he was tired out, and dropped down with his back against the door, and said he would rest a minute and then kill me. He put his knife under him, and pretty soon he dozed off.

Huckleberry Finn
Mark Twain

Social problems

In previous times, it was said that marijuana smoking was a 'crime without a victim', but even then no one would have called alcoholism a victimless 'crime'. The victims of alcoholism are legion: spouse, children, other relatives, bosses, fellow workers, pedestrians, drivers, police, judges, physicians who get called late at night, taxpayers who often pick up the bill for treatment, and other innocent and not so innocent people who cross the alcoholic's path. Here are some telling statistics.

1. Before drugs became a major problem in the USA and other countries, the average city policemen spent half of his time dealing with alcohol-related offences. Nearly half of the men and women in prison were alcoholic or, at any rate, heavy drinkers. Most murderers were drinking at the time they committed a murder, and so were most of the victims, although how many would be considered alcoholic is uncertain. Today, US jails and prisons are full of people arrested for crimes involving illicit drugs. Many of them are also heavy drinkers. The relative contributions of drugs and alcohol to their criminal activities become difficult to separate. This also applies to the problems mentioned below.

2. Between 20 and 30 percent of male psychiatric admissions are alcoholic or have alcohol-related problems. About a quarter of the men admitted to general hospital wards for medical treatment have alcohol-related problems.

3. Industry loses huge amounts of money every year because of absenteeism and work inefficiency related to alcoholism. Monday morning and Friday afternoon absenteeism, at least partly attributable to alcoholism, is so common that both industry and union officials have considered a four-day working week (whereupon Tuesday morning or Thursday afternoon absenteeism would probably become common).

4. Alcoholics are about twice as likely to be divorced as non-alcoholics.

5. Alcoholics have a death rate twice as high as that of non-alcoholics. The most common causes, aside from medical diseases, are accidents and suicides. There are an estimated 20 000 deaths a year from alcohol-related automobile accidents in the USA, accounting for approximately 40 percent of all traffic fatalities. Studies indicate that most of the drinking drivers are not just social drinkers coming home from a Christmas party but serious problem drinkers—alcoholics by most definitions. About one out of four suicides in the USA is an alcoholic, usually a man over 35.

6. According to the US Department of Justice (1996), 36 percent of all convicted offenders were drinking alcohol at the time of their offense, and one in five violent crimes was committed by a perpetrator who was perceived (by the victim) to be under the influence of alcohol.

In 2003, the Cabinet Office Strategy Unit Alcohol Project estimated the economic cost of alcohol misuse in Great Britain at up to £20 billion per year. The cost to industry due to lost productivity and illness was estimated at £6.7 billion, and the cost to the National Health Service of alcohol-related injuries and illness was estimated at up to £1.7 billion a year. Alcohol misuse was responsible for approximately 150 000 hospital admissions and linked to between 15 000 and 22 000 premature deaths per year. The cost of alcohol-related crime was estimated at £7.3 billion per year, with nearly half of all violent crimes involving a perpetrator who had been drinking.

Alcohol-related problems

In one survey of American drinkers, 18 per cent had experienced at least one problem from drinking in their lifetime. They were also, at some point in their life, heavy drinkers, meaning that they drank almost every day and had six or more drinks on at least one occasion per week. Half of the heavy drinkers (9 percent) stopped being heavy drinkers for several years and had no further difficulty with alcohol.

Should these former heavy drinkers who later drank normally be called alcoholics? Whether to do so is partly a matter of definition, but also reflects often intense, almost religious, views of what alcoholism is and is not. There is no question that many people who have *minor* and *infrequent* problems from drinking can control their drinking. An alcoholic, by definition, is a person with *severe* alcohol problems who cannot control his drinking. More about this later.

Following the order in which problems for the alcoholic were described, here are some comments about these problems as experienced by non-alcoholics.

It is not true to say that non-alcoholics do not think much about alcohol. Social drinkers (as they are sometimes called) may have excellent control over the amount they drink and still look forward to a preprandial aperitif (and miss it when they do not get one). They look forward to what used to be called 'getting drunk and having fun' on New Year's Eve. Many college students look forward to the beers they plan to consume after taking a tough examination. It is still socially acceptable, in most parts of society, to celebrate weddings, birthdays, anniversaries, and reunions with an old friend with a drink (often not limited to one drink). Georges Simenon had this to say about drinking in the USA (and he was not talking solely about alcoholics).

… [Americans experience] an almost permanent state in which one is dominated by alcohol, whether during the hours one is drinking, or during the hours when one is impatiently waiting to drink, almost as painfully as a drug addict waits for his injection … If one has never known this experience, it is difficult to understand American life. Not that everyone drinks, in the

> sense in which my mother used the word, but because it is part of private and public life, of folklore, you might say, as is proved by the large, more or less untranslatable vocabulary, most often in slang, that relates to drink ...
>
> All of life is colored by it. New York, for example, seems made to be seen in this state, and then it is an extraordinary New York and, strange as it may seem, comradely.
>
> The crowds cease to be anonymous; the bars cease to be ordinary ill-lit places, the taxi-drivers complaining or menacing people. It is the same place for all big American cities. Los Angeles, San Francisco, Boston ... From one end of the country to the other there exists a freemasonry of alcoholics ...
>
> Georges Simenon

Simenon's description may have fitted the USA better in the 1920s and 1950s (when he wrote it) than it does today. Attitudes toward drinking have changed in the past 50 years, with drunkenness much less tolerated. Still, bars continue to outnumber churches (and even grocery stores) in American cities, despite the legal perils of embarking on the highway after drinking as little as two drinks (the legal limit for intoxication in the USA has been dropped to 0.08 percent nationally, which two drinks will produce in some people). Beer commercials continue to dominate sports commercials, even if the beer today is sometimes non-alcoholic beer. Many Americans are at least somewhat preoccupied with alcohol, even though they would not be described as alcoholic.

The non-alcoholic heavy drinker also often lies to himself—or at least to his doctor. Physicians are convinced that, most often with regard to controlling a patient's weight or ruling out a possible cause for a medical condition, drinkers, when asked, minimize the amount of alcohol they drink. People who drink even moderately may have concerns that their drinking may not be so moderate after all—that it may indeed lead to serious drinking—but they do not want to give up all alcohol if they can help it, and so they reduce the amount they drink. (In alcoholics, this would be called 'denial'.)

Does the moderate drinker with an occasional problem from drinking experience guilt? Sometimes. Simenon said, 'In the United States I learned shame. For they are ashamed. Everyone is ashamed. I was ashamed like the rest'. Any drinker who has been charged with drunken driving because he had three or four drinks on one occasion (perhaps more than he had ever consumed previously) knows the feeling. Anyone who has had a hangover probably knows the feeling. The novelist Kingsley Amis said that hangovers take two forms: physical and metaphysical. He considered the metaphysical part (the guilt) far more distressing than the nausea and headache.

More than a third of middle-class American men have experienced at least one alcoholic blackout (as defined above) by the age of 20. It has been said that having memory lapse (blackout) while drinking as a young person means that the person is doomed to become alcoholic later in life. This has been shown to be untrue. Most people who have experienced one or even several blackouts do not become alcoholics. On the other had, alcoholics have many blackouts, particularly as they get older.

Even a single drink will make some people feel depressed. After several drinks they may feel profoundly depressed, especially the next morning. This has been called *alcohol-induced dysphoria*. It only happens to a minority of people, but it is one reason why some people give up alcohol entirely. It just isn't worth it. Of course, the phenomenon can also have the opposite effect if the person turns to drinking in an attempt to suppress these feelings.

Incidentally, alcohol-induced dysphoria appears to occur most often in people who have a susceptibility to depression when not drinking. Manic-depressives, for example, tend to drink less when depressed than when not depressed probably because alcohol loses its interest for people who are depressed or they have found that even a little alcohol makes them feel more depressed, particularly the next morning. Manic-depressives may be more likely to drink during manic phases of the disease, possibly in an attempt to level out the 'high'.

As for medical problems from drinking, even small amounts of alcohol will cause heartburn or diarrhea in some people, and may worsen a stomach or duodenal ulcer if one is already present. Drinkers who develop a particular type of cirrhosis are usually described as alcoholic, but there is some disagreement about this. Some studies have reported the occurrence of cirrhosis in people who staunchly defend themselves as moderate drinkers. Doctors' skepticism about drinking histories, born of hard experience, may result in an over-diagnosis of alcoholism in moderate drinkers. Pancreatitis can certainly occur in drinkers who consume far less than does the typical alcoholic.

Some experts believe that even modest amounts of alcohol consumed on a regular basis may cause subtle impairment of brain functioning that can become permanent. Most experts believe that drinkers who limit their alcohol to a drink or two per day are probably in no danger of brain damage.

Moderate drinkers who drink immoderately on some occasions are as suscep-tible to sexual dysfunction as the hard-drinking alcoholic.

Even light drinkers often believe that a drink or two at night takes the edge off their effectiveness the next day or may contribute to migraine headache (which it probably does) or a downright unwillingness to show up for work, at least until noon. This may be all in the imagination, as the saying goes, but many people believe it.

Finally, moderate use of alcohol in some drinkers may produce social prob-lems. Some people may physically abuse their spouse or children but would never think of doing so if they had not had two or three drinks (usually it takes more). Two or three drinks may produce just the amount of courage needed to rob a shopkeeper. Two or three drinks may not mix well with prescrip-tion tranquilizers or sleeping pills or non-prescription cold medication. These combinations may produce driving errors and bad social judgment that would not have occurred with one ingredient alone.

7

The course

➡ Key points

♦ The natural history or natural course of alcoholism is not as clear as some might believe. Who is selected for study and what is studied will define the picture of what happens to alcoholic individuals over time, even when they are given treatment.

♦ As a result, calling alcoholism a disease also remains a source of controversy. Professionals who do not think of alcoholism as a medical disease often view it as learned behavior that can be unlearned. The debate continues. But fortunately, compared with decades ago, fewer and fewer people today believe that alcoholism is 'just' a moral weakness or personal deficiency.

♦ More people recover from alcohol abuse than alcohol dependency. Alcoholic drinking waxes and wanes over time for most people who drink unwisely. Some alcoholic individuals seem to recover from their addiction and can drink normally, but most cannot.

♦ The power of the addictive cycle is remarkably strong; it can consume the life of a person and those who care about him.

What happens to people who are called 'alcoholic' or are said to suffer from alcohol abuse or alcohol dependence? What happens to them if they stop drinking? What happens if they continue to drink? Can alcoholics learn to drink responsibly? Can the family or loved ones do something to stop alcoholism? How well does treatment work? At first glance, these are really straightforward questions that should have straightforward answers. These questions have been studied for more than seven decades, and hundreds of millions of dollars have been spent on research. But the answers to these questions are not so straightforward. They depend on what group is studied, how long they are studied, and what is studied. There is no simple or single answer to the question: 'What happens to alcoholics?' There are still debates about what alcoholism is, how it should be defined, how well treatment works, and what is meant by recovery. Depending on how one answers these questions, the answers to the question 'What happens to alcoholics?' will differ.

Answers to the simple questions 'What happens to alcoholics?' and 'What works with alcoholics?' are surprisingly complex. It is like the story of the six blind men who come to quite different conclusions about what an elephant is after each one has examined a different part of the animal with their hands. About a half a century ago, almost every program created to treat alcoholics in the USA had a very famous poster hanging on its wall. This wall poster illustrated a graph first presented by E.M. Jellinek (many consider Dr Jellinek as the father of empirical research into the nature and causes of alcoholism). Jellinek's graph showed a large U-shaped curve. The stages that all alcoholics were supposed to pass through until they 'hit bottom' were listed on the left-hand side of the curve. Hitting bottom was represented by the lowest part of the U-shape. These stages into drunken helplessness included events like blackouts, lost jobs, and separation from family until, finally, the individual drinker was so consumed by alcoholism that all he did was 'drink his life away', regardless of its horrible consequences. Then at the very bottom of the U-shape, hitting bottom, a very fat black horizontal line was drawn to the right with an arrow at the end pointing to the word DEATH that was written in even fatter and blacker letters. The word 'death' was often followed by a skull and crossbones.

This famous poster announced for all to see the moment they entered into the treatment program that the course of alcoholism was progressively malignant and inevitably resulted in death unless the individual stopped drinking altogether. On the right-hand side of the U-shape were listed the stages of recovery after the individual completely stopped drinking. It was assumed that once the individual stopped drinking, he or she would return to a full, happy, and productive life. This view of the natural history or natural course of alcoholism dominated the thinking of both treatment personnel and the general public for many years. It turns out that this view of the natural course of alcoholism was incorrect. A small percentage of alcoholics do become progressively worse and do die homeless and alone if they do not stop drinking. However, the majority do not follow this course. Some alcoholic drinkers do live full and productive lives when they stop drinking, but many continue to have significant social and emotional problems even when alcohol is no longer part of their lives.

So, how did those catastrophic ideas become so embedded in the public consciousness? The U-shaped curve was generated from a survey of recovering alcoholics who belonged to Alcoholics Anonymous (AA). All were once severely alcohol dependent and all later stopped drinking after they 'hit their bottom'. The idea that alcoholic individuals are likely to die if they do not stop drinking was a fantasy based on little evidence at the time that this famous poster was made. Even Jellinek himself recognized that the information contained in the poster was misleading.

What causes people to disagree so much about what happens to alcoholics? The answer is that the results of outcome studies are entirely dependent upon the group of alcoholics that are studied in the first place. Outcomes also vary dramatically depending to the length of time that alcoholics are studied and what definitions are used to identify alcoholism and especially recovery from alcoholism. The results of studies that begin with a severely and chronically addicted group of alcoholics selected from an inpatient treatment setting look quite different from the results of population studies that begin with large numbers of people selected from the general public or recruited from advertisements placed in the newspaper. The findings of a one month or three month follow-up study of alcoholic drinkers will give a much more optimistic picture of the course of alcoholism than follow-up studies performed five, ten, or more years later. The course of alcoholism defined only by how much and how often a group of people drink in the past month or year will not look the same as the course of alcoholism defined by the number of physical, emotional, or behavioral problems that are associated with drinking over long periods of time. Recovery rates from alcoholism will also look very different if total abstinence from alcohol is used as the definition of recovery rather than a reduction in the volume of drinking or the number of problems associated with drinking over a given period of time.

Two older studies illustrate why it is so difficult to come up with a nice simple straightforward answer to the question: 'What happens to alcoholic drinkers?' One study was performed in a metropolitan area and focused on homeless alcoholic men who had at least five contacts with the police for drinking-related offenses in the previous five years. In contrast, the other study started with a group of highly skilled professionally trained individuals. All these professionally trained people were practicing their profession at the time they were treated. All were receiving inpatient treatment in a private hospital as a stipulation to continue practicing their generally well-paid professions. Most had families and were considered successful by others. All of the patients in this second study would be carefully monitored by a state authority once they returned to their work.

When complete abstinence from alcohol was used as a measure of recovery, *none* of the homeless alcoholic sample achieved abstinence after five years and many of these men had died. The number of serious medical problems found in this previously homeless group was extraordinary compared with the professionally trained group. What happened to the professionally trained group after five years? Over 85 percent of the professionally trained alcoholic subjects were able to achieve abstinence after five years, and 99 percent successfully went back to work for some period of time. Some of the homeless men drank less and some found regular housing but, over all, this group did very poorly. Most of the high-profile private treatment centers for alcoholism claim 'success' in well over two-thirds of their clients as measured by abstaining from any alcohol. In contrast, abstinence is typically reported to occur in only about a third of the alcoholic patients being treated in a public facility.

In a study of two very different groups of men over 60 years, George Valliant found more alcoholic drinking in the socially disadvantaged group compared with the advantaged group. He also found less alcoholic drinking over time among both groups, but the disadvantaged group continued to show more alcoholism than the advantaged group even after 60 years.

What all this means is that the course of alcoholism is highly variable. It differs widely across individuals and different groups of individuals. This level of variability fuels the strongly argued debates about the true nature of alcoholism. Is it a disease or is it a learned behavior? Should alcoholism be classified into all-or-none categories or be defined as a dimension or continuum like blood pressure? What does recovery from alcoholism really mean: total abstinence from alcohol consumption or controlled drinking without problems? Until an agreement is reached about these very fundamental definitions, debates will continue in the study of alcoholism.

Even so, the fact is that the constellation of drinking behaviors and drinking effects that are commonly referred to as alcoholism do indeed reflect a very serious condition that can destroy the life of an individual. The costs are enormous. It is a condition (we would say a disease) that begins relatively early in life. It typically waxes and wanes, worsens and improves over time, as alcoholic drinkers age. It tends to lessen in severity toward the end of life if people live long enough. It creates great suffering for individuals, those that love them, and the communities in which they live. The World Health Organization reports that alcoholism is one of the leading causes of mortality and morbidity through out the world.

The good news is that, for most, alcoholism is not a hopeless unchangeable condition. The bad news is that there is no single type of treatment or treatment program that can be depended upon to stop or modify alcoholic drinking for everyone. Dozens of different kinds of treatments have been tried. Most seem to benefit some alcoholics, but treatment overall seems to do little to change the natural course of alcoholic drinking in different groups. The good news is that many things seem to work in helping alcoholics stop or reduce abusive drinking as long as they stick to it and are willing to make a commitment to change. It is the 'sticking to it' that seems to make the critical difference in what will work and with whom, whether that involves daily AA meetings, religious/spiritual awakening, individual counseling, family therapy, medication, or some combination of these.

A lot is known about certain events and personal characteristics that seem to be associated with alcoholic drinking. This information is useful because it is interesting, it is sometimes helpful in treating individuals with alcoholism, and it can lead to a discussion about possible ways for society to reduce or prevent alcoholic drinking. It must be kept in mind that something that is related to, or associated with, a condition such as alcoholism is *not* the same as a cause. It is called a correlation.

People make the mistake over and over again in thinking that an association is the same as a cause. It might be. But, it might not be. For example, men all over the world are more likely to develop a problem with alcohol than women, even though overall rates of alcoholism vary widely from country to country. This does not mean that being male 'causes' alcoholism. It just means that gender is strongly associated with alcoholism. It is a risk factor for alcoholism, not a cause. It could be that something associated with being female is protective. Another example: countries vary widely in their rates of alcoholism, but this does not mean that a country 'causes' alcoholism. Studies from all over the world indicate that as people get older, they tend to drink less and less. This is also true of alcoholics as a group. This finding does not mean that youth 'causes' alcoholism, just that alcoholism, as presently defined, tends to peak in the middle and early twenties, with women peaking a little later than men.

Almost all studies indicate that alcoholics have a higher mortality rate than moderate drinkers, but that total abstainers also have a higher mortality rate. There have been many attempts to explain this remarkable finding. One plausible explanation is that abstainers are abstaining because of poor health and its attendant increased risk of mortality. Other possible explanations are insufficiently validated to justify any comment on them. Some protection against mortality is most commonly reported for red wine drinkers, but there are also studies reporting that this is also true for alcohol in any form *in moderation*.

It seems that alcohol decreases the chances of blood clotting and may also reduce arteriosclerosis, as noted earlier.

Disease, again

Diseases tend to have a predictable course or 'natural history'—to progress or terminate in more or less predictable ways if not modified by treatment. In the USA, alcoholism is widely considered a disease despite the fact that its course over long periods of time can vary dramatically across different groups of alcoholic drinkers. The American Medical Association has taken this position. Others disagree. Many opponents of the disease concept believe that 'problem drinking' or 'heavy drinking' (they avoid the medically and AA-tainted word 'alcoholism') is a form of learned behavior and should be treated, not as a disease with drugs or even psychotherapy, but as a learned behavior that can be unlearned by appropriate techniques, usually applied by psychologists.

Professionals who reject the disease model accept the idea that dependence (physical and psychological) occurs, but believe there are *degrees of dependence* rather than an all-or-nothing phenomenon called alcoholism. They are probably correct. When talking about extreme dependence, they describe something close to what is called alcoholism, but avoid the word. They believe that even extremely dependent drinkers can be treated by modifying what is basically learned behavior. They are distressed when heavy drinkers are viewed as 'helpless victims of a disease', which may only serve as an excuse for continued drinking. This point of view is cogently presented in a book by Hubert Fingarette called *Heavy drinking: the myth of alcoholism as a disease* (University of California Press, 1988) and continued in a more recent book called *Mapping responsibility: choice, guilt, punishment and other perspectives* (Open Court, 2004).

It is with regard to the course of the illness (which opponents do not consider an illness) or the natural history that one finds the strongest disagreement. Advocates of the learning theory approach believe that even severely dependent drinkers can learn to drink normally, at least in many cases. Their focus is on 'harm reduction' rather than abstinence. Here the *disease–non-disease* conflict clashes head on. Extremely dependent drinkers, called alcoholics by most American therapists, are admonished that they can never drink normally, and to try to drink will ultimately end in disaster. The belief that total abstinence from alcohol is the only practical goal of treatment is based in part on the philosophy of AA, and is also held by most American physicians and many physicians in other countries.

There is no controversy about whether most non-dependent 'heavy drinkers' could drink in moderation if they decided to do so, and surely no one would call heavy drinking in itself a disease. Most individuals who abuse alcohol do recover over time, possibly because they are getting older or possibly because of other life changes, such as getting married or getting a job, which are associated with a marked drop in alcohol consumption.

What is controversial is whether severely dependent heavy drinkers—alcoholics—can ever return to normal drinking. It is feasible for non-dependent drinkers, many of whom go on to become controlled problem-free drinkers with or without professional help. Those who do not succeed, despite professional help, are usually the most dependent drinkers. However, it is important to keep in mind that frequent drinking and episodic heavy drinking are strong predictors for developing more severe problems in the future. Heavy drinking is also a risk factor for a whole host of medical and social problems, as stated before. The US Department of Health and Human Services suggests that a safe drinking limit for men is no more than 2 ounces of alcohol per day. Safe drinking limits for women are less than 1 ounce per day. Some would say that these standards are too lax and some would say that they are too strict. The debate continues.

Concerning the word 'dependence'—for a long time dependence referred to a physical state (where a person must use alcohol to avoid withdrawal symptoms) or a psychological state (where the person's life revolves around seeking and drinking alcohol at the expense of other activities). At present, the word 'dependence' does not require physical symptoms. Instead, the word is used to reflect a relatively large number of negative consequences caused by drinking.

This change in the definition of dependence will also change how the course of alcoholism plays out. Whether there is a clear line between non-dependent heavy drinking and dependent alcohol drinking is not known. Some would say that 'true' alcoholism does not lie on a continuum but is a separate medical diagnostic entity. Others would say that the evidence points to a continuum of heavy or problem drinking. In order to really say that alcoholism is or is not a separate and distinct clinical entity, not a continuum, one would need a separate and distinct way of identifying alcoholism without relying on the volume consumed or the number of problems experienced. We do not have that type of independent measurement currently available. Maybe we will some day, and then many of the controversies in the study of alcoholism will disappear.

Natural history

When does alcoholism begin? Fixing the onset of a chronic condition is difficult. In cancer, when does the first cell become malignant? When does the first
plaque begin to form in heart disease? Cancer and heart disease can usually
be diagnosed only after they are much farther advanced, and the same is true
of alcoholism. With some alcoholics, alcoholism seems to start with the first
drink, but this is only recognizable in retrospect, after looking back in time.

Nevertheless, the condition tends to develop at certain ages, progresses in a
more or less predictable manner, and terminates in more or less predictable
ways. 'More or less' is an important qualifier, as there is much variation. Men
and women vary, as well as different races and nationalities.

The 'typical' white male alcoholic begins drinking heavily in his late teens
or early twenties, drinks more and more throughout his twenties, starts having serious problems in his thirties, is hospitalized for drinking (if ever) in
his middle or late thirties, and is clearly identified by himself and others as
alcoholic—a man who cannot drink without trouble—between the ages of 40
and 50.

With rare exceptions, men do not first become alcoholic after 45. There is an
'age of risk' for alcoholism, as for most illness, and if a man has no symptoms
of alcoholism by his late forties, he probably will develop none.

As discussed earlier, the illness may end by death from suicide, accident, or
medical illness–or by cessation of drinking. In the view of many experts, few
alcoholics can return to normal or non-harmful drinking.

Patterns of drinking are variable between people and over time. It is a mistake
to associate one particular pattern exclusively with 'alcoholism'. Even severe
alcoholics can stop drinking abusively for a time, but their chances of doing so
for long periods are frighteningly small. Many types of alcoholism exist, and
many individuals who do not conform to traditional alcoholism stereotypes
still have serious drinking problems. One drink does not invariably lead to
a binge; a person may drink moderately for a long time before his drinking
begins to interfere with his health or social functioning.

The diversity in drinking patterns explains the current emphasis on problems as the basis for diagnosing alcoholism. Modern researchers have tried
to identify and validate subgroups of alcoholics. Identification of subgroups
should reduce some of the striking clinical diversity found when large groups
of alcoholic people are studied for many years. Reducing the amount of

clinical diversity should result in more accurate predictions and, hopefully, more effective treatments. It might also provide some information about cause.

Many different methods of subtyping alcoholic drinkers have been developed. No single one is completely accepted. Many methods of subtyping alcoholics use impulsive and antisocial behaviors as distinguishing characteristics. Alcoholics who show a lot of impulsive and antisocial behavior in early life usually begin to abuse alcohol at a younger age and have a more severe course over time. Another method of subtyping alcoholics depends on the presence or absence of alcoholic drinking among close biological relatives. Family-history-positive alcoholics also seem to drink addictively at an earlier age and also have poorer outcome than alcoholic drinkers without a positive family history of alcoholism. Not surprisingly, these two ways of subtyping alcoholic drinkers are highly correlated. In fact, our studies show that all the major methods of subtyping or subgrouping alcoholics are highly related. We are not sure what this means; perhaps there is some common factor that has yet to be identified.

Before 1970, most alcoholics in treatment centers could be described as 'pure' alcoholics. If they also used drugs, it was to relieve anxiety and insomnia—often caused by alcohol—or to find a substitute for alcohol that was less destructive. Nevertheless, alcohol remained their 'drug of choice'. Since drug abuse became so widespread in subsequent years, more and more alcoholics are also drug abusers, and their 'drug of choice' may be cocaine or opiates rather than alcohol. Assuming that these individuals drink or use drugs in order to achieve some pleasurable state (or to escape some less comfortable state), they presumably select for the particular drug or drug combination that is best suited to produce the desired effect. The polydrug phenomenon is complex and too recent to be fully understood; it has certainly complicated treatment and altered the natural history of uncomplicated alcoholism in ways that are still poorly understood.

Recent studies have examined 'spontaneous remission' or 'natural recovery' in more detail than previously. The results are very 'sobering'. They suggest that as people get older, they tend to drink less. This is true of normal drinkers, problem drinkers, and alcoholic drinkers. However, alcoholic drinkers continue to drink the most, problem drinkers a little less, and normal drinkers even less or they stop altogether. When asked, older people will often say that drinking alcohol fails to make them 'feel good' or that drinking alcohol makes them feel 'sick'. We do not know the mechanism for this, but it seems that old rats also lower their consumption, compared with younger rats, when offered alcohol. Older rats also show more adverse behavioral effects to alcohol than younger rats at the same dose. As well as aging, other experiences seem to be associated with spontaneous remission or natural recovery. Graduating from college, getting married, having a child, or joining a religious group seem to reduce consumption and the problems that accompany drinking. However, these effects are usually small and usually parallel getting older. The 'sobering' aspect of spontaneous remission or natural recovery is that these frequently profound changes in a person's life occur outside the context of treatment or professional help. For those people who do not spontaneously stop drinking or cannot moderate their drinking, the addictive cycle can become an over-powering reality.

Addictive cycle

> Live moderately because great pleasures rarely go unpunished.
>
> Puritan moral

Any ultimate explanation of alcoholism or alcohol dependence must account for two features of the illness: *loss of control* and *relapse*. Loss of control refers to the alcoholic's inability to stop drinking once he starts. Relapse is the return to heavy drinking even after a period of sobriety. This is one of the true mysteries of addictions.

Why, after months or years of abstinence, does the smoker smoke again, the junkie shoot up again, the alcoholic fall off the wagon? We are not sure. It is a great puzzle that seems to reflect the interplay between inherited and environ-mental factors—the combined effect of biology and learning. What is known about the brain's role in these processes is discussed in Chapter 12.

It appears that some people experience more pleasure, or glow, from alcohol than others. This effect may be partly determined by heredity. The pleasure is short-lived and, in some people more than others, it is often followed by feelings of discomfort. The *degree* of pleasure and the degree of discomfort caused by alcohol may also be determined by heredity. Alcoholics learn that the discomfort they experience after drinking has a simple remedy—another drink. Thus the alcoholic drinks for two reasons: to achieve pleasure and to relieve discomfort. In the beginning, the discomfort that alcohol relieves for a time may be anxiety, depression, anger, shyness, boredom, self-hatred, or sim-ply the fear of not belonging. In older people, alcohol can temporarily relieve pain or promote sleep. But, once alcohol has become established as a way to experience pleasure and reduce discomfort, another process takes over.

The same substance that produces the happy feeling also begins to produce an unhappy feeling. Alcohol is then required both to restore the one and to abolish the other. Nothing abolishes the unhappy feeling quite as effectively as the drug that produced it. This unhappy feeling is sometimes referred to as *withdrawal*, but the term 'withdrawal' is not a particularly good word to refer to what happens when an addicted person stops drinking. Withdrawal usually refers to the profound bodily effects that accompany a sudden large drop of alcohol in the blood. These bodily effects are short-lived, but go hand in hand with a strong negative psychological effect that can last for months and even years after an alcoholic stops drinking.

The unhappy feeling is called craving. The alcoholic will try anything to relieve craving—a chocolate bar, sex, tranquilizers, jogging, or prayer—but has learned that only alcohol gives complete and immediate relief. After a time, the alcoholic drinks more to overcome the unpleasant effect of abstinence than to attain the pleasant effects of alcohol. This is another great mystery addressed in Chapter 12. Over time the addicted person may drink alcohol to 'feel normal' and avoid the discomfort of craving and may no longer drink for the pleasure it once gave them.

What triggers this craving?

Leaving aside free will, relapse can partly be explained by something called *stimulus generalization*. The term refers to the fact that things remind people of other things. For the drinker, the hands of a watch pointing to 5 p.m. (the stimulus) may remind him that, for years, he always had a drink at 5 p.m. (the generalization), and so he drinks. Acts of drinking become embedded in a maze of reminders or *cues*. Every drinker has his own reminders, but there are common themes. Food, sex, holidays, football games, fishing, travel—all have nothing intrinsically to do with drinking but all commonly become associated with drinking and are powerful reminders. Physical feelings (hunger, fatigue) become reminders. Moods (nostalgia, sadness, elation) become reminders. In short, anything can be a reminder and *remain* a reminder long after a person has stopped drinking.

Reminders may lead to relapse. One day, unexpectedly, the 'recovered' alcoholic is flooded with reminders. It is 5 p.m. on Christmas Eve (which is also his birthday). The boss had been complaining and he missed lunch. His alimony check to his wife bounced, but he learns he has just won the Irish sweepstake. Suddenly he has an incredible thirst. As he passes a pub, a strong west wind blows him through the door—and a relapse occurs. This is an extreme example. The relapse trigger may be subtle.

For any alcoholic, there may be several or a whole battery of critical cues or signals. By the rule of generalization, any critical cue can spread like the tentacles of a vine over a whole range of analogs, and this may account for the growing frequency of bouts, or for the development of a pattern of continuous inebriation. An exaggerated example is the man who goes out and gets drunk every time his mother-in-law gives him a certain wall-eyed look. After a while he has to get drunk whenever any woman gives him that look. In either case, the relapsing alcoholic probably will not be able to say later why he started drinking again. Stimulus generalization is probably not the whole story. But it seems to explain a lot. It is, also, a useful idea to build a relapse prevention program for people who are determined to stop or moderate their drinking.

Mark Keller

8

Women and alcohol

> ## ➜ Key points
>
> ◆ Although alcoholism is more prevalent among men, the disease may represent a more serious syndrome in women.
>
> ◆ Women tend to develop alcoholism later in life than men, but the disease course as well as the progression of alcohol-related health complications seems to occur at a faster rate.
>
> ◆ Gender differences in the manifestation of alcoholism are likely to result from combined inherited biological, social, environmental, and psychological factors.
>
> ◆ Fetal alcohol spectrum disorder (FASD) is a cluster of symptoms that may be found in infants and children who were exposed to alcohol before birth.
>
> ◆ The most devastating effects of FASD are associated with damage to the developing baby's brain which can result in persistent mental and behavioral problems.

Most studies of alcoholism and alcohol-related problems have historically dealt with men. One reason for this is that men are more often alcoholic than women and it is easy to find male alcoholics if you want to do a study. As previously stated, the US government estimates that approximately 7 percent of men and 3 percent of women, nationally, meet criteria for alcohol abuse, and 5 percent of men and 2 percent of women meet full criteria for alcohol dependence. Attention to gender issues in research has shifted somewhat in recent years and numerous studies are now devoted to female alcohol problems. For example, after many years of all-male twin studies, a study of female twins was undertaken in the early 1990s. Even in women, heredity apparently plays a major role in alcoholism, although the specific relationship is not well defined.

Some studies have provided interesting distinctions between male and female drinkers. The most talked about distinction arises from the woman's ability to be pregnant. It is now clear that drinking and pregnancy do not mix. The specific effects of alcohol on the fetus will be discussed later.

 Facts

♦ Women who become alcoholic tend to develop the disease at an older age. As noted earlier, if men are not alcoholic by their mid-forties, they probably will not become alcoholic. This is less true of women.

♦ Women alcoholics are more likely than men alcoholics to have a depressive illness, and the onset of depressive illness is more likely to precede the development of alcoholic disease.

♦ In addition to depression, alcohol use disorders often co-occur with eating disorders, especially bulimia nervosa. This relationship exists for both genders, but eating disorders are generally more common among women than men.

♦ Alcoholism in women seems to be more serious than in men. Women are harder to treat and stay sober for briefer intervals than men. Woman also appear to progress from first use to significant alcohol problems faster than men, a phenomenon called telescoping.

The relatively low frequency of alcoholism among women has been the source of a great deal of conjecture and controversy among alcohol researchers. However, years of scientific study has solidly and consistently shown that alcoholism, worldwide, occurs two to three times more often in men than in women. It is not known whether this difference is due to psychosocial or biological attributes, although one might predict that both factors are involved. Differences in the onset and course of alcoholism in women are also somewhat of a mystery and are in need of substantially more research emphasis.

More attention has been given to differences in the health effects of alcohol on women than men. Less attention has been focused on the predictors or possible causes of alcoholism in women. It is clear that women have more medical complications——particularly liver disease——from heavy alcohol use than men and experience them after fewer years of drinking. They may also become intoxicated on smaller amounts of alcohol. If women do indeed become intoxicated on smaller amounts of alcohol (and certainly this does not apply to all women), it is partially because women are generally smaller than men. Smaller people tend to get drunk on less alcohol simply because less is required to fill a small space. Two other factors may be important: women in general have more body fat than men; alcohol is less soluble in fat than in water and so the alcohol concentration in the blood and other watery parts of the body is higher in women after drinking equal amounts.

Recent studies also show that women achieve higher levels of blood alcohol than men do after consuming the same amount because, in women, more alcohol passes directly into the small intestine where it is absorbed rapidly into the bloodstream. The reason why women metabolize less alcohol in the stomach appears to be because an enzyme that breaks down alcohol is less active in the stomachs of women than in the stomachs of men.

 Facts

◆ Women are more susceptible to alcohol-related physical health problems at lower exposure levels than men. This includes a faster progression of brain damage in women. This effect is probably related to biological factors that increase the levels of alcohol in the bloodstream of women compared with men at equal doses.

◆ Heavy drinking is associated with a significantly greater risk of death in women than men. One study estimated that heavy drinking (defined as six or more drinks per day) increased a women's risk of death by 160 percent compared with light drinking (defined as more than one drink per month but less than one drink per day). Similar drinking patterns increased mortality in men by 40 percent.

◆ Alcohol use is associated with an increased rate of breast cancer in women. As mentioned previously (Chapter 4), this effect may result from alcohol-related deficiencies in folic acid (vitamin B_9) since taking the vitamin appears to eliminate the association.

There is the factor of expectation. Americans have long believed that women cannot 'hold' their drink as well as men. As a result many of an older generation held the view that women should not drink at all. Prior to the early 1900s, most bars in the USA were by custom restricted to men, and if a woman ventured into any bar alone she was often automatically assumed to be a prostitute.

Attitudes toward drinking by women appear to have been different in the UK and the wine- and beer-drinking countries of Western Europe. There is the common idea today that women are drinking more than ever, and perhaps this is true in the USA, but it is not so in every country. In 1892 the *British Medical Journal* was 'appalled' by the increase of drunkenness among women in England as well as in 'other parts of the world'. The number of women convicted of drunkenness had doubled in 10 years, rising from about 5000 to 10 000 in 1884. In Ireland the 'champion female inebriate had been arrested over 700 times, and is yet less than 40 years old'. The *Journal* said that whereas formerly men alcoholics outnumbered women alcoholics by seven to one, by 1892 the ratio was three to one. The age of the offenders ranged from 12 to 60. Female alcoholism was called a 'national shame'. Alcoholic women were said to represent all classes and conditions of society. The editor believed that this increase of inebriety extended to all civilized countries, but conceded that he had no evidence for this. (There were not many statistics in those days.)

The *Journal of the American Medical Association* responded to its British counterpart in 1892 by saying that there was no problem with female alcoholism in the USA.

It may be safely asserted that the American woman cannot constitutionally use any form of alcohol as her foreign sisters use it. She has more acute nervous organization, and the brain centers are more unstable; the surroundings are full of psychological factors that keep up a certain nerve tension, which antagonizes the sudden increase in the heart's action from alcohol. The brain suffers from the strain of alcohol, which gives no pleasure. The American women of all classes want rest, not increased excitement; hence they seek this more naturally in narcotics. [There was an epidemic of unregulated opium use by both sexes in the USA and UK in the nineteenth century.]

The American editor urged that the British should stop arresting women alcoholics and pleaded that alcoholism was a disease in both sexes and the domain of medicine not the law:

The time is coming when the medical profession will teach the world the causes and remedies of the great and widespread evil of the century.'

Journal of the American Medical Association

This was written in 1892. One hears the same words today. The 'causes and remedies' have remained elusive.

What is the situation today? We certainly know much more about gender effects in drinking than we did 100 years ago.

It remains true that there are more men alcoholics than women alcoholics. Some believe the gap is closing, but there is no direct evidence for this.[1] The best current estimate of the sex ratio for alcoholism in the USA is 3:1 (male:female).

With 'liberation' has come an increase in women drinkers. In secondary schools as many girls now drink as boys. More women are now also engaging in after-work cocktail hours and work-related social events. Such changing roles and social norms have been associated with increased alcohol use among women.

But has there been an increase in alcohol problems among women? Probably not. Less than 10 percent of women are heavy drinkers, meaning that they drink almost every day and get intoxicated perhaps several times a month. Between 20 and 40 percent of men fall in this category, with young men more likely than older men to be heavy drinkers.

Because more girls are drinking than apparently ever before it is commonly assumed that the rate of heavy drinking and alcoholism will automatically increase in women. This may not occur since more women than men are physiologically intolerant of alcohol; after a modest amount of alcohol, more women experience dizziness, headache, nausea, or a sense of simply having enough. Since this 'protection' is physiological and probably genetically determined, presumably it will not disappear even though more secondary school-girls and professional women are drinking more often.

 Facts

- Women who are part of a cohesive family unit with a successful marital partnership and multiple roles (wife, mother, employee) are less likely to become alcoholics. This may or may not be related to the beneficial effects of a stable spousal relationship.

- Drinking patterns in women tend to follow the level of drinking in their husband or male partner. It is unclear whether women with drinking problems 'seek out' men with drinking problems, a phenomenon referred to as 'assortative mating', or if alcoholic men simply encourage heavy drinking in their partners.

> ◆ Being sexually abused is a risk factor for the development of several psychological disorders, including alcoholism, in men and women. Women victims of sexual abuse (as adults or children) are more likely to develop alcohol use problems.
>
> ◆ Women who drink alcohol increase their risk of physical assault or victimization, particularly by a male partner. In a study of 1160 female victims, most cases of physical assault occurred when both the man and the woman had been drinking.

Aside from obvious gender differences in physiological tolerance toward the effects of alcohol, it is also quite clear, stereotypes aside, that the brains of men and women are, quite simply, 'wired' differently. Emerging technologies are only beginning to define the neurobiological differences between the sexes and are a long way away from explaining the influence of these differences on drinking habits. However, it is highly likely that many of the observed differences in the manifestation of alcohol problems in men and women are rooted in the particular responsiveness of the male versus the female brain to the effects of alcohol.

 Fact

> ◆ A recent study has concluded that black women and white women engage in heavy drinking in about equal numbers. Black women seem to have fewer alcohol-related social and personal problems than white women but may carry a greater share of alcohol-related health problems. Hispanic women are more likely to drink less or abstain, although more moderate and heavy drinking is reported among young American-born Hispanic women.

Fetal alcohol syndrome

Women have been told for a long time that they should not drink during pregnancy. The idea goes back at least to biblical times. In Judges 13:7 an angel tells Samson's mother: 'Behold, thou shall conceive and bear a son: and now drink no wine or strong drink'.

In early Carthage bridal couples were forbidden to drink for fear of producing a defective child. According to Aristotle, 'Foolish, drunken and harebrained women most often bring forth children like unto themselves, morose and languid'.

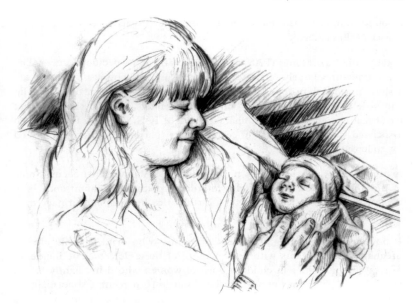

Figure 8.1 'Precious future.' Artwork by Lorie Gavulic.

In 1834 a report to the House of Commons said: 'Infants of alcoholic mothers often have a starved, shrivelled and imperfect look'.

The biblical injunction does not make it clear why pregnant women should not drink. The concern may have been that the child would become alcoholic. Plutarch said that 'drunkards beget drunkards', reflecting a belief held well into the twentieth century that traits and habits acquired by parents would be passed along to the offspring. There was also the theological view that the sins of the fathers, and no doubt the mothers, would be passed on.

Convincing evidence has emerged over the last several decades that pregnant women should not drink, or drink much, for another reason: heavy drinking may produce fetal abnormalities.

What exactly is fetal alcohol syndrome?

The syndrome was first described with any precision in an obscure French gynecological journal in 1968 and again, with much more publicity, in 1972 by two Seattle pediatricians. These reports led to a fervent search for the syndrome in children of drinking women. After many conferences, large amounts of money spent on research, and passionate disagreement, a kind of consensus has emerged.

Fetal alcohol syndrome (FAS) has specific and non-specific features. The specific features largely relate to the head. An FAS baby has a small head, a short nose, a thin upper lip, an indistinct groove between the upper lip and nose (called the philtrum), small eye openings, and flat cheeks. These facial features are considered characteristic of FAS, although they are also associated with maternal use of certain drugs (particularly those prescribed for epilepsy).

A multitude of other features not specific to FAS may also occur. Some of these include low birth-weight, retarded growth as an infant and child, mental retardation, heart murmurs, birthmarks, hernias, and urinary tract abnormalities.

It now appears that 30–50 percent of women who drink 'heavily' during pregnancy have infants with one or more of these defects. The incidence of fetal abnormalities in children born of women who drink lightly or not at all during pregnancy appears to be about 5–10 percent. (Abnormality is used here in a broad sense, referring to anything from a birthmark to missing limbs.)

The term 'fetal alcohol effects' has been suggested to describe these non-specific fetal abnormalities. It has become increasingly clear that the specific facial characteristics of FAS are fairly rare and may occur in only the most severe cases. Fetal alcohol spectrum disorder (FASD) is a more general term referring to any set of disorders that may result from drinking during pregnancy. It is estimated that FAS occurs in one in every 1000 live births, while FASD may occur as often as one in every 100 births.

While FAS is most notably reflected in the *faces* of affected offspring, perhaps the most serious manifestations of FASD involve changes in the *brain*. These changes can produce major psychological problems such as:

- hyperactivity

- attention problems

- cognitive deficits

- social and behavioral problems

- learning and memory problems

◆ IQ deficits

◆ verbal and language problems.

Additionally, for various reasons FASD individuals appear to be more likely to have a multitude of psychiatric disorders such as attention deficit–hyperactivity disorder, depression, schizophrenia, disorders related to conduct, in particular, such as criminal behavior, sexual deviance, and alcohol and/or substance misuse. In fact, FASD-affected individuals, perhaps by virtue of being born to mothers who drank, possess many of the same risk factors that have been found to predict the development of alcoholism.

The precise cause of FASD has remained somewhat controversial, and it is still unclear what level of alcohol consumption causes injury. The only clear proof of pathology comes from studies in animals. These studies have determined with some certainty that, in animals, fetal exposure to alcohol directly interferes with brain development. Prenatal alcohol exposure of rats and mice disrupts communication between developing neurons and alters the migratory paths of new neurons, leading to structural changes in several specific brain regions.[2] These abnormalities correspond to brain changes observed in human FASD. However, confirmation of these findings in humans is more complicated than it may outwardly appear. A large number of competing and confounding factors have prevented a conclusive assessment of the specific effects of alcohol on the human fetus.

Most studies of human FASD examine babies born either to mothers known to consume alcohol during pregnancy or, more often, to alcoholic mothers with unknown if not *presumed* alcohol consumption during pregnancy. There are several important factors for consideration in these comparisons. First, alcoholic women are often heavy smokers and often use other drugs suspected of causing fetal abnormalities. In addition, the overall health of alcoholic women is typically poorer. They tend to have poor nutrition and may be deficient in important nutrients such as folic acid and thiamine which are critical for fetal brain development. Moreover, alcoholic women generally have a different lifestyle from that of non-alcoholic women, which undoubtedly factors into the development of their babies.

At least 70 percent of alcoholic women smoke cigarettes. Women who smoke cigarettes tend to have small babies, whether they drink or not, so perhaps cigarette smoking and not alcohol is responsible for the small babies born to alcoholic women. Because non-smoking alcoholic women are rare, this is a difficult question to answer. Studies suggest that alcohol abuse and cigarette smoking contribute independently to small size of the newborn. The best estimate at present is that alcohol abuse approximately doubles the risk of birth of a small infant, whether the mother smokes or not.

Another factor to consider is heredity. Birth defects run in families. So does alcoholism. Is it possible that in some instances a common genetic predisposition explains both? There is little evidence for this one way or the other. However, some reports about twins suggest that this explanation may not be far fetched. Sometimes one twin shows signs of FAS and the other does not; if alcohol is solely responsible, this should not happen.

Timing is crucial in fetal development. Even brief exposures to a virus or drug early in pregnancy can determine whether or not a limb is formed; birth size relates mainly to events occurring in the last two or three months of fetal development. Considering the complexity of the systems involved, it is not surprising that FASD has come to describe such a broad range of effects. How much a pregnant woman can drink without risk to her child is not known and perhaps never will be.

Obviously there is a great deal of uncertainty about FASD and how often it occurs. To what extent should women modify their usual drinking patterns because of concern about FASD? Many women spontaneously reduce their alcohol intake during pregnancy because alcohol makes them ill. Should they reduce their intake to zero?

Some years ago, investigators of FAS made the following recommendation.

Observations of human babies and of experimentally treated animals have made it clear that a mother's heavy drinking can severely damage her unborn child. We do not know the exact amount or timing of drinking that causes these effects. We cannot say whether there is a safe amount of drinking or whether there is a safe time during pregnancy. We do know that heavy drinking can be damaging. Women should therefore be especially cautious about drinking during pregnancy and when they are likely to be pregnant.

Most authorities still believe that this is good advice. Of course, to be absolutely safe, pregnant women should not drink at all.

There are thousands of women in AA and in alcoholism treatment facilities who have apparently normal children. Many more children of problem-drinking mothers will have to be studied before FASD can be defined with certainty. Meanwhile, caution is obviously the wisest course.

The question as to whether pregnant women should drink raises another: Should women drink while breast-feeding? There is certainly alcohol in the milk. If the mother is intoxicated while breast-feeding, the infant may become intoxicated. No one knows for certain whether this will harm the infant. Newborns are in a vulnerable and rapidly changing stage of development. One would expect them to be especially sensitive to any environmental insult, including alcohol. Not drinking for a few hours preceding nursing, and during nursing, is undoubtedly the safest course.

Section 3

Understanding alcoholism

First the man takes a drink, then the drink takes a drink, then the drink takes the man.

Japanese proverb

Understanding alcohol

9

Risk factors

> ## → Key points
>
> ◆ There are a number of so-called 'risk factors' which appear to predict the development of alcoholism. The most important of these are male gender, a family history of drug abuse or alcoholism, and the presence of other mental problems.
>
> ◆ Researchers believe that inherited or biological factors are the greatest contributors to the development of alcoholism. These biological factors include certain childhood behaviors which are influenced by heredity and biology.
>
> ◆ Alcoholism is probably the result of combined influences of biological, interpersonal, and environmental factors.

Whether alcoholism is something that is learned and therefore can be unlearned, or like a cancer where the victim is powerless to shrink the tumor without help, the fact remains that there is no scientifically acceptable explanation of why some people develop problems from alcohol and most do not. Billions of dollars and several decades of research have been dedicated to solving this mystery. While the specific cause or causes of alcoholism are still unknown, a number of so-called 'risk factors' have been identified which appear to influence the development of drinking problems. Used in the classical epidemiological sense, a risk factor should both predate and predict the development of alcoholism. The terminology is used more liberally in this discussion and also includes factors that are correlated, or commonly co-occur, with alcoholism but do not necessarily predate the development of alcoholism. Such factors are not true risk factors for alcoholism because it is not always possible to determine whether the factor *contributed to* or *resulted from* the drinking problem. Nevertheless, these influences are an important consideration when evaluating who may be at risk.

The strongest risk factors or predictors of alcoholism appear to be the result of inherited or biological attributes. Three have been linked to alcoholism: male gender, a family history of drug or alcohol problems, and the presence of additional mental or psychiatric disorders.

Gender

Almost all studies confirm the higher prevalence of alcoholism in men than in women. Alcohol-related disorders are considerably more common in men than in women—usually greater than a 3:1 ratio. Throughout history and in every culture studied, men outnumber women in becoming alcoholic. This suggests that cultural factors may not be as important as genetic or physiological factors in explaining the difference between rates of male and female alcoholism. Emerging evidence from brain imaging technology has identified clear neurobiological differences between the sexes which may contribute to the observed gender differences in risk for alcoholism.

Family history

Alcoholism runs in families. Children of alcoholics become alcoholic about four times more often than children of non-alcoholics. There is evidence that they become alcoholic whether or not they are raised by their alcoholic parent. (This evidence is examined in Chapter 11.) Other studies have found clear behavioral and physiological abnormalities in the children of alcoholics that are associated with an increased risk for alcoholism later in life. These include impulsivity, poor self-control, and abnormal brain responses to activating stimuli. Although a precise gene has never been identified, it is widely accepted among alcoholism researchers that genetic factors are a major contributor to the vulnerability to developing alcoholism. Alcoholism in the family is probably the strongest predictor of alcoholism occurring in a particular individual. The more close biological relatives with alcoholism, the greater is the vulnerability. However, it is important to remember that not all children of alcoholics become alcoholic. Even though their chances of developing alcoholism are greater than individuals with no alcoholic relatives, it is still more likely that individuals with a family history of alcoholism will not develop alcoholism.

Psychiatric problems

Alcoholism commonly coexists with other psychiatric problems, and, like alcoholism, psychiatric problems tend to run in families of alcoholics. The treatment and management of psychiatric conditions are commonly complicated by the presence of co-occurring substance abuse problems. Alcohol abuse, in particular, is a factor in a large number of admissions to psychiatric hospitals.

Several specific psychiatric disorders are particularly common among alcoholics. Depression and anxiety are the most common. Some of these disorders undoubtedly result from or are exacerbated by alcohol abuse, and therefore are not true 'risk factors'. However, there is increasing evidence that certain childhood behavioral problems—deregulation, dyscontrol, and deviance—may predate exposure to alcohol. These characteristics are referred to as endophenotypes and are believed to influence, directly or indirectly, vulnerability to the development of alcohol problems. Attention deficit–hyperactivity disorder and childhood conduct disorder are both considered to be risk factors for the development of alcoholism. The relationship between alcoholism and other mental disorders is discussed in more detail in Chapter 10.

 Myth

Addictive personality

There is a popular misconception that the development of alcoholism emerges from a particular addictive personality type. The so-called 'addictive personality' was drawn from personality characteristics observed in recovering alcoholics and drug addicts. These observations on a very select sample were strongly influenced by drug effects as well as the aftereffects of drug withdrawal, and do not represent characteristics which contribute to the development of alcoholism. The public acceptance of the addictive personality persona may also stem from lay observations of clustered comorbid mental problems, such as attention deficit–hyperactivity disorder, in individuals with alcoholism. While certain personality *disorders* may be more common among alcoholics, research has dispelled the idea of a specific addictive personality type. Alcoholism can be and is associated with all kinds of personalities. The search for the addictive personality really was more of an effort to find something to 'blame' for a person's inability or unwillingness to stop drinking abusively.

Other possible influences (correlates)

Age

Age is another important biological attribute that appears to influence the development of alcoholism. Alcoholism in men usually develops in the teens, twenties, and thirties. Men who are not clearly alcoholic by their mid-forties are unlikely to become alcoholic later, using the definition for alcoholism in Chapter 5. It is not uncommon for women to develop alcoholism in their forties; but people over 65 rarely become alcoholic, regardless of sex. This does not mean that alcohol may not adversely affect them in later years, and occasionally it does.

Drinking in adolescence

Some researchers have suggested that teenagers may be especially sensitive to developing an alcohol problem because of the biological changes associated with their particular developmental stage. Adolescence encompasses a major growth phase in human development. As described in Chapter 2, excessive use of alcohol during this period may have profound and lasting effects on the individual. However, it is still not clear whether adolescent exposure to alcohol specifically increases the **risk** of developing alcoholism or other addictions. Based upon what is currently known about the responses of adolescents to alcohol, several theories have been proposed.

◆ It has been suggested that adolescents may require more alcohol than adults to achieve the same level of euphoria or 'high' which might encourage escalated alcohol use.

◆ Adolescents might also experience fewer adverse physical effects from drinking than adults, which would be expected to reduce some of the negative consequences associated with alcohol intoxication.

◆ Other theories suggest that developmentally determined behavioral traits may impair impulse control and judgment in teenagers, thereby encouraging alcohol or drug experimentation.

◆ Newer theories suggest that enhanced adaptability or 'neural plasticity' that is associated with brain growth in adolescents may strengthen brain connections linked to alcohol use experiences.[1]

While these theories are all very interesting, it is important to note that there is little direct scientific evidence to support any one of them at present. These models are consistent with studies in animals, but their direct relevance to human adolescents is not known. Risk factors for adolescent drinking problems encompass sociocultural considerations such as regulation of drinking, availability, parental behavior and drinking patterns, the influence and drinking habits of siblings and peers, and personality traits, particularly those indicating low self-regulation and passive beliefs about alcohol use. The factors that predict adolescent problem drinking are similar to those that predict alcohol problems in general and may also be influenced by heredity.

Studies have shown that people who start drinking at a younger age do have a poorer disease course, but this may have little to do with the age that they began to drink. It may be that individuals *predisposed* to alcoholism, possibly due to inherited factors, simply seek out or are exposed to alcohol at an earlier age. More research is needed to address these questions specifically.

Race

Alcoholism occurs in all races and ethnic groups worldwide. Rates of alcoholism among blacks, whites, and Hispanics in the USA appear to be similar. Some groups, such as Irish and Native Americans, have more alcoholism, while Jewish and Asian Americans seem to be at lower risk. It is not clear how many social/cultural versus biological influences contribute to these relationships. The prevalence of alcoholism among Native Americans varies dramatically by tribe and is believed to be strongly influenced by genetic factors. However, Native Americans living on reservations are also subject to additional stressors caused by their generally poor living conditions.

Social and environmental factors

Is biology in itself sufficient to doom one to a life of struggle with alcohol? Undoubtedly, some level of exposure to alcohol is necessary. Psychologists have long abandoned the notion of the so-called 'latent' alcoholic. You must drink alcohol to become an alcoholic; however, just how much exposure is necessary before problems emerge varies between individuals.

Environmental factors do contribute to the development of alcoholism. Specific factors related to the **availability** of alcohol are important. Cultures and countries where the use of alcohol is forbidden or access is strictly controlled appear to have lower rates of alcoholism. Psychosocial stressors, such as poverty, abuse, and neglect, are associated with increased rates of alcoholism. Certain **occupations**, such as bartender, may be associated with more or less alcohol use; although it is not clear whether particular occupations contribute to the development of alcoholism. Alcoholics may simply select positions where the hours and work conditions are favorable to drinking. Conceivably, bartenders become bartenders because of the availability of alcohol on the job.

As for nationality, global estimates of alcoholism rates are difficult to interpret since reporting and diagnostic definitions tend to vary from one country to the next. According to the World Health Organization (2002), the rates of alcohol dependence in reporting countries varied from 0.2 to 12 percent. The rate of alcohol dependence was highest for Poland, Brazil, and Peru at 11–12 percent, and lowest for Egypt, Nigeria, and Singapore at 0.2–0.7 percent. The USA fell in the middle of this range at 7 percent, while the UK was slightly lower (5 percent).

The development of alcoholism appears to be based upon an accumulation of multiple biological, interpersonal, and social factors. Biological factors influence the perception of alcohol's effects as well as the development of personality characteristics needed for the appropriate regulation of drinking behavior. Interpersonal and social influences determine the number of life-stresses experienced by the individual, and social factors influence the level of alcohol exposure. The respective roles of these influences must be defined, independently and in combination, to permit the development of effective strategies for treatment and recovery.

10

Alcoholism and co-occurring mental illnesses (dual diagnosis)

> ### → Key points

- Alcoholism is associated with a number of different mental illnesses such as mood and anxiety disorders, schizophrenia, and some personality disorders. Sometimes, this combination of illnesses is called 'dual diagnosis'.

- Many alcoholics suffer from two, three, or four additional co-occurring mental illnesses which makes the term 'dual diagnosis' somewhat misleading and confusing.

- Alcoholics with one or more co-occurring mental illnesses tend to have more difficulty stopping or reducing their drinking. On the whole, the quality of life is much poorer among alcoholics with co-occurring mental illnesses.

Comorbid illness

When the first edition of *Alcoholism: the facts* was published in 1981, an active and sometimes acrimonious debate was swirling about among research scientists and clinicians. The question under debate was: Is alcoholism mostly a stand-alone mental illness that is largely unrelated to other mental illness? Or, is alcoholism commonly associated with other mental illness like depression, bipolar disorder, schizophrenia, anxiety disorder, and even the personality disorders?

It is an important question because the answers *should* have a major impact on treatments that are offered and research that is performed. The debate hinges on something that is called the *base rate*. A base rate is an estimate of how many people have, or have ever had, a certain condition in a particular group. Usually, the reference group is the general population. In mental health, base rates estimate how many people in the general population currently suffer from, or have ever suffered from, the more common mental illnesses such as mood and anxiety disorders as well as drug and alcohol abuse/dependence. These estimates can be broken down by gender, age, race, or any other selected individual feature if enough people are studied. The early debate focused on the base rates then available for the different mental illnesses. Some researchers said: 'Yes, people suffering from alcoholism do have an unusually large number of other co-occurring mental illnesses when compared with the general population'. Their opponents said: 'No, the results supporting a greater prevalence of additional mental illness among alcohol-dependent people is an artifact caused by the physiological effects of consuming large amounts of alcohol over long periods of time'. For example, they argued that the very use of alcohol in large quantities over time might cause depression or anxiety symptoms in individuals with alcoholism. It was often a heated debate.

That debate has pretty well been settled now, although subtle variations of the argument are still bouncing around. A very strong consensus about this issue has been reached worldwide. It is now widely agreed that alcoholism is *highly associated with elevated rates* of a large group of mental illnesses. The strength of that association will depend, not surprisingly, on the particular group of alcoholics that are studied in the first place (see Chapter 7). The relationship between alcoholism and other mental illnesses is strongest among people with the more severe form of alcoholism, for example alcoholics requiring inpatient treatment. More co-occurring mental illness is found among hospitalized alcoholics than among individuals recruited from the community. More co-occurring mental illness is found among people with alcohol dependence than with alcohol abuse. The meaning of this association is yet another question. The significance of the elevated rates of co-occurring mental illness with alcoholism continues to be argued.

Very often the term *comorbidity* is used to indicate the co-occurrence of alcoholism and at least one other mental illness. Comorbidity is a useful term: it simply means the presence of two or more illnesses, regardless of when they started or how severe they become. The term 'comorbidity' does not imply that one condition causes the other; sometimes a causal relationship exists between the two illnesses, and sometimes it does not. Even so, the term comorbidity is still a little too imprecise for some specialists, but it is a good word to keep in mind. The words 'co-occurring' and 'comorbidity' are used interchangeably in this book. Some people use the term 'dual diagnosis' to refer to the co-occurrence of alcoholism with at least one other *non*-substance abuse mental disorder. We prefer to avoid this label. The term 'dual diagnosis' is even more imprecise and a little misleading to those just learning about this interesting clinical phenomenon. Dual diagnosis implies only one other mental disorder co-occurring with the alcoholism. Two are common.

Implications for course and treatment

The clinical significance of co-occurring or comorbid mental illnesses with alcoholism is not fully understood. Questions like the following still exist.

- Does alcoholism cause the other mental illness?

- Do other mental illnesses cause the alcoholism?

- Does one illness make the others worse?

- Does the recovery from one illness make the recovery from, or management of, the other easier?

- Is it better to treat the co-occurring mental illness and alcoholism separately or together?

- If one of the comorbid mental illnesses is successfully treated, what is the impact on the other comorbid mental illnesses?

- What happens (what is the course?) to people with alcoholism and another mental illness?

- Does the type of comorbid mental illness make a difference on the drinking outcomes? Or, on quality of life outcomes?

Much is unknown about the relationship between alcoholism and other comorbid or co-occurring mental illnesses, but a fair amount is known. In the scientific literature, co-occurring mental illnesses are usually called psychiatric disorders. The terms mental illness and psychiatric disorder are used interchangeably in this chapter. When we write about mental illness or psychiatric disorders, we refer to the definitions found in the the *Diagnostic and statistical manual of mental disorders, version 4* (DSM-IV, TR) published in 2000. This manual, a diagnostic guide for professionals in the mental health field, provides straightforward definitional criteria for most of the mental illnesses.

Alcoholics identified in large community samples typically have less comorbid illness than alcoholics who are receiving treatment for their drinking problem in a hospital. The pattern of co-occurring mental illnesses is different for men and women alcoholics. As true for non-substance-abusing samples, depression and anxiety disorder occur more often in women than men alcoholics while drug abuse and antisocial personality disorder occur more often in men than women alcoholics. These differences among the two genders are typically found all over the world and clearly do not depend upon the presence of substance abuse or substance dependence.

One half or more alcoholics in treatment are likely to have another comorbid psychiatric illness, if the clinician takes the time to look for it. Unfortunately, providers often do not look for psychiatric comorbidity. All too often, symptoms suggestive of another mental illness are discounted as one more problem caused by the excessive drinking. Sometimes this is true, but sometimes it is not. This sort of 'blind spot' can occur for a number of reasons. Sometimes treatment providers are not adequately trained to recognize, identify, and appreciate separately the effects of alcoholic drinking from the symptoms of other mental illnesses. Some 'stand-alone' alcohol treatment programs choose to ignore the existence of psychiatric comorbidity because they do not have the ability to treat them adequately. And sometimes comorbidity is ignored because the idea is a newer one and traditional ways of thinking are sometimes very hard to change.

If comorbid psychiatric illnesses are simply due to the effects of excessive drinking, the onset of the co-occurring mental illness would, necessarily, begin *after* the alcoholism begins. On the other hand, if the alcoholism developed because of an attempt to 'medicate' pre-existing psychiatric illnesses, the onset of the comorbid mental illnesses would occur *before* the alcoholism begins. It turns out that both of these statements are sometimes true. A third of comorbid alcoholic people do report that problematic drinking began well before any other psychiatric illness. In another third of people who suffer from both, alcoholic drinking occurs at a later age than other comorbid mental illness, and in another third, alcoholic drinking and other co-occurring mental illnesses started at about the same time.

Does it really make any difference?

Many people once thought it did. It was argued that depression, even clinical depression, beginning *after* the onset of alcoholism is different from the clinical depression that is experienced before the onset of alcoholism. Clinical depression first experienced after the alcoholism began was called 'secondary depression' (secondary refers to the temporal order of the first occurrence of the two illnesses). Clinical depression that preceded the onset of alcoholism was called 'primary depression'. Some argued that these were two different kinds of depressions. There are few data to support this view. In one study, the primary–secondary distinction made no difference to the outcomes of hospitalized male alcoholics. The primary–secondary distinction did not differentiate family history of mental illnesses or response to treatment or the presence of a third or fourth co-occurring psychiatric disorder.

Today, the primary–secondary distinction is generally viewed with disfavor mainly because we now know so much more about the true extent of the entire range of psychiatric comorbidity found among alcoholic individuals. Initial studies of comorbidity focused almost exclusively on clinical depression among alcoholics because depression was so common. However, once the full range of mental disorders was systematically studied in large groups of people with alcoholism, the usefulness of the primary–secondary distinctions diminished. It simply made little clinical sense to think about primary versus secondary schizophrenia or primary versus secondary bipolar disorder or primary versus secondary panic disorder. With the notable exception of the dementias, most major psychiatric illnesses begin at a relatively early age, and some begin earlier than others. Psychiatric illnesses such as social phobia, attention deficit disorder, antisocial personality disorder, and mild mental retardation begin very early in life and are more likely to precede the onset of alcoholism. Others that begin a little later in life (for example, in the twenties) are more likely to follow the onset of alcohol drinking. Therefore, the temporal order of the onset of alcoholism and another co-occurring psychiatric disorder may be an artifact with little real clinical relevance—a function of the usual lifetime emergence of the various illnesses rather than any meaningful causal association.

If the primary–secondary distinction is not particularly relevant to the clinical treatment of comorbid illnesses with alcoholism, then what is?

The number and type of co-occurring mental illnesses are especially important and relevant considerations. As the number of comorbid psychiatric disorders increases among alcoholics, the probability of recovery from any one lessens. As the number of comorbid disorders increases among alcoholics, the likelihood of an early age of onset of alcoholic drinking is also increased. Early-onset alcoholism is usually associated with a greater severity of illness than late-onset alcoholism. As the amount of psychiatric comorbidity increases, the more probable it is that close biological relatives will also have suffered from a host of mental illnesses, including higher rates of familial alcoholism. Finally, the childhood environments of alcoholic individuals with co-occurring mental illnesses tend to be more unstable and dysfunctional than the childhood environments of individuals who suffer from only alcoholism, and, generally speaking, the more dysfunctional the childhood environment, the more severe the later alcohol problems are likely to be.

The type (or types) of co-occurring psychiatric disorder also influences the course and outcome of alcoholism treatment. The type (or types) of comorbid psychiatric disorder is also associated with the family history of mental disorders and childhood environment. If the comorbid psychiatric illness is associated with especially poor clinical and social outcomes, then alcoholics with that comorbid illness will generally do less well over time than individuals who suffer from alcoholism only or alcoholic individuals who suffer from a comorbid illness that typically has a more favorable outcome. The course for people diagnosed with schizophrenia and alcoholism is typically much worse than the course for people with alcoholism and a phobia, regardless of the amount of alcohol consumed. Thus the type (or types) of co-occurring illness plays a major role in what happens to alcoholics. The type (or types) of co-occurring psychiatric illness would also be expected to play a major role in what treatments(s) are offered to each individual. Unfortunately, this is not always true.

People who suffer from alcoholism along with another comorbid psychiatric disorder do not do as well in life as people who suffer from alcoholism only. They are more likely to relapse. They experience more medical, social, and legal problems, and they do not respond as well to conventional treatment approaches. Psychiatric comorbidity is common; in some treatment samples, it is the norm.

How can this phenomenon be ignored by so many?

There are many historical and political reasons why greater efforts and resources are not devoted to the treatment of people who suffer from alcoholism and another mental illness. These reasons include turf wars between professions, poorly integrated funding sources at the national and state levels, and separate administrative structures for mental health and substance abuse that span conflicting insurance policies and governmental agencies. There are still mental health providers and programs who do not want to treat substance abuse, and there are still substance abuse treatment providers who do not want to treat mental illness, just as there are physicians who treat cancer and others who treat diabetes.

Probably, the strongest reason why more attention is not given to the so-called 'dually diagnosed' individual is the lack of effective treatments for the combination. At present, there are no *unique* treatments that are specific to particular comorbid combinations. Instead, most alcoholics who also suffer from a co-occurring mental illness receive treatments that were originally developed to treat either alcoholism or the comorbid mental disorder, not both. The majority of treatment programs currently available focus on either the alcoholism or the co-occurring disorder(s). When both the alcoholism and the co-occurring disorder(s) are the focus of treatment, the clinician must apply separate treatments to each disorder. Treatments designed originally for sufferers of alcoholism are combined with treatments originally designed for sufferers of the comorbid disorders. This is true for pharmacological as well as psychosocial treatments. These 'grafted' programs are limited in their effectiveness. Antidepressant medication does not always work as well for the depression of alcoholics as for the depression that stands alone. Schizophrenics with alcoholism do not necessarily respond as well to antipsychotic medications as those with schizophrenia alone. Bipolar mania in alcoholics is less successfully treated with mood stabilizers than bipolar mania alone. The popular 12-step Alcoholics Anonymous (AA) program does not appear to work as well for the alcoholic with a comorbid psychiatric disorder.

The most carefully studied comorbid combination is the combination of alcoholism with a mood disorder like major depression or bipolar illness. Controlled pharmacologic studies suggest that the treatment of comorbid mood disorders with medication is not effective in treating either the co-occurring mood disorder or the alcoholism. Clinicians who continue to use antidepressants and mood-stabilizing medications with alcoholics are convinced that these agents do sometimes help. It is hard to be sure. A real problem in treating 'dual diagnosis' patients is that they tend to be extremely non-compliant with treatments of all kinds. These patients are even more non-compliant with treatment than the alcohol-only patients, who are notoriously non-compliant.

When more effective and specific treatments become available for alcoholic sufferers with comorbid psychiatric disorders, we suspect that many of the current barriers will rapidly disappear. One bright spot on the horizon is the development of Dual Recovery Anonymous (DRA) which was founded by Tim Hamilton and his friends in Kansas. Tim has first-hand knowledge of what it is like to suffer from a serious substance abuse problem (i.e. drugs and alcohol) combined with other comorbid psychiatric (and medical) disorders. He has been sober for over 20 years, but continues to battle symptoms of four different psychiatric conditions and several medical ones. Tim was, and still is, a great supporter of AA. He believes that AA saved his life. Over time, Tim realized that the traditional 12-step approach of AA did not address other causes of his suffering that were the product of comorbid psychiatric conditions. He recognized that, for some people, the traditional AA approach was not enough. Tim started over from scratch. With the help of others, he slowly created DRA which now has chapters all over the world. Tim and his friends ultimately developed a unique and highly specific 12-step self-help group approach which addressed the combined effects of substance abuse and one or more co-occurring psychiatric disorders. Simply blending or combining existing treatments is not enough. Genetic, familial, developmental, and environmental studies as well as carefully performed treatment outcome studies are needed in order to better serve the alcoholic who also suffers from a co-occurring mental illness. In the end, individualized treatment strategies may work the best.

11

Heredity

We are as days and have our parents for our yesterdays.

Samuel Butler

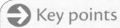 Key points

- It has been well established throughout history that alcoholism runs in families.

- Familial alcoholism typically can be distinguished from non-familial alcoholism by its tendency to have a more severe and highly malignant course which usually begins at a younger age and is more likely to be associated with the presence of other psychiatric conditions.

- The passage of alcoholism among family members is believed to be strongly influenced by genetic factors.

- There does not appear to be a single gene for alcoholism; rather, scientists favor a model in which multiple genes in combination add to the vulnerability of developing alcoholism in varying degrees.

Alcoholism runs in families. This has been known for centuries. Plutarch said that 'Drunkards beget drunkards'. Aristotle said that 'Harebrained and drunken women have harebrained and drunken children'. The nineteenth-century medical and religious literature is replete with references to the familial aspect of alcoholism. Clergymen blamed the 'sins of the father' for the transmission of alcoholism from generation to generation. Doctors attributed the transmission to deleterious effects of alcohol on the sperm or egg, a consequence of parental imbibing at the time of conception.

Numerous studies in the twentieth century document the familial nature of alcoholism. About 25 percent of the sons and 5–10 percent of the daughters of alcoholics become alcoholics. The prevalence of alcoholism in the general population is around 5 percent in men and 1 percent or less in women. Having alcoholism 'in the family' increases one's chances of becoming alcoholic by a factor of four or five to one.

Not everything that runs in families is inherited. Speaking French runs in families and is not inherited. It is often hard to separate 'nature' from 'nurture' in conditions that run in families—the same people who provide our genes usually bring us up.

One way of distinguishing between the influence of heredity and environment is to compare identical and fraternal twins. Characteristics controlled by heredity should coexist in identical twins (since they share the same genes) and differ in fraternal twins (whose genes are shared only to the extent that siblings share genes). In other words, assuming that large noses are inherited, both identical twins should have large noses but one fraternal twin may have a large nose and the other have a small nose. If alcoholism is influenced by heredity, both identical twins would develop the illness more often than would both fraternal twins. Does this happen?

There have been many studies of alcoholism in which identical twins were compared with fraternal twins. In general, identical twins more often had similar drinking habits, alcohol-related problems, and alcoholism than did fraternal twins, indicating a genetic influence. However, heredity could not totally explain alcoholism in the twins. In some pairs of identical twins, one twin was alcoholic and the other was not. If genes completely controlled the development of alcoholism, both identical twins should *always* be alcoholic.

Of course, no one expected that this would happen. Obviously, environmental factors, such as cultural attitudes and the availability of alcohol, are important. In few inherited disorders is there 100 percent correspondence between the occurrences of the illness in both identical twins.

Another way of determining whether heredity influences the development of a familial disorder is to study people who have been adopted. In the case of non-family adoptions, individuals are raised by different people than those who provided their genes.

The original author of this book, Don Goodwin, and colleagues from America and Denmark conducted the first large-scale study of alcoholism in adoptees. It was conducted in Denmark because of easy access to adoption records.

First studied was a group of young Danish men who had a biological parent hospitalized for alcoholism but had little or no contact with their parents because they were adopted away early in life and raised by adoptive parents. Eighteen percent of these men were also alcoholic at a young age (before 30). The rate of alcoholism in this group was four times greater than was found in a comparison group of adoptees of the same age and sex who did not have an alcoholic biological parent. In this study, the presence of alcoholism in the biological parents clearly distinguished the adopted sons of alcoholics from the adopted sons of non-alcoholics. Alcoholism-related problems in people who were not alcoholic did not show evidence of a genetic influence.

Also studied were the sons of alcoholics who were raised by their alcoholic parents. This group had the same rate of alcoholism as did the sons of alcoholics who were adopted by non-relatives in infancy and had no exposure to their alcoholic parent.

In addition, the Danish–American research group studied daughters of alcoholics, both those raised by their alcoholic biological parents and those adopted away in infancy and raised by non-alcoholic adoptive parents. Both groups of daughters had high rates of alcoholism compared with the general population. A group of adopted women without known alcoholism in their biological parents also had a high rate of alcoholism, raising the possibility that adoption itself in some way promoted alcoholism in women.

Two other adoption studies were subsequently performed by others, one in Sweden and the other in Iowa. Both studies initially produced the same results as the Danish studies: an increased prevalence of alcoholism in adopted-away children of alcoholics. Later analysis of the Swedish data and expansion of the Iowa study detected environmental factors influencing alcoholism in the adoptees (especially heavy drinking in the adoptive parents) and an association of antisocial personality disorder and alcoholism in male adoptees. The three sets of studies differed widely in methodology (one was purely a record study), but they continued to find evidence of genetic factors in alcoholism.

The concept of 'familial alcoholism' has developed from these studies. This differs from 'non-familial' alcoholism in having the following features.

◆ There is a family history of alcoholism.

◆ The alcoholism develops at an early age (usually by the mid-twenties in males).

◆ The alcoholism is severe, often requiring treatment.

◆ Having alcoholism in the family also appears to coincide with increased risk of other psychiatric disorders such as antisocial personality disorder.

Subsequent studies have reported increases in anxiety and mood disorders in addition to antisocial personality disorder and drug abuse in adopted-away children of alcoholics. It should be noted that antisocial characteristics are typically manifested in men, while women are more likely to develop depression. In both cases, the psychiatric condition may predate the development of alcoholism. The precise genetic influence of an inherited risk for alcoholism on the risk of developing other psychiatric conditions is not entirely clear. An important consideration in this equation is the presence or absence of other psychiatric syndromes in the parents which may contribute in separate or additive ways.

The idea that alcoholism can be subdivided into two types, familial and non-familial, has generated some new research findings.

It seems that about half of alcoholics have alcoholism in the family. Of those who have alcoholism in the family, about 90 per cent have *two* or more relatives who are alcoholic. (This is also true of other illnesses influenced by heredity, such as breast cancer and late-onset diabetes.) The younger the alcoholic at the time of diagnosis, the more likely it is that there will be alcoholism in the family. Familial alcoholism tends to be particularly severe.

If alcoholism in some individuals is influenced by heredity, what is inherited? No one knows, but over the course of several decades the US government has invested large amounts of money in the search for biochemical mechanisms which might explain how the risk for developing alcoholism is transmitted from generation to generation.

Alcohol produces changes in neurotransmitter activity. Neurotransmitters are chemicals that transmit signals from one brain cell to other brain cells. Inherited abnormalities in the functioning of several different neurotransmitter systems have been suggested to influence the risk of developing alcoholism. Of these, the neurotransmitters dopamine, serotonin, gamma-aminobutyric acid (GABA), and glutamate, as well as several neuropeptides[1] such as the opioid peptides and neuropeptide Y, all appear to play a role in the addiction process. Biological molecules from each of these neurotransmitter systems have been proposed as 'candidates' for specific genes that may increase the risk of alcoholism. Of particular interest are the molecular targets of the neurotransmitter dopamine, especially the D_2 dopamine receptor, which appears to be altered in some alcoholics and their relatives.

The ultimate jackpot in alcoholism research would be the identification of a single gene, or group of genes, that influences drinking behavior. Unfortunately, it is widely believed by molecular biologists that this will not be possible. The most popular 'genetic' model, at the moment, offers a 'multigenetic' explanation for the inheritance of alcoholism. This model suggests that alcoholism results from an accumulation of effects from *many different* genetic factors. The rationale for this theory is that the complexity of the behavioral symptoms associated with alcoholism cannot be explained simply by an effect on only one gene or a small cluster of genes.

Genetic linkage studies of alcoholics have indeed identified a number of different genes which appear to impart vulnerability toward the development of alcoholism. Most of these genes affect the biological response of the brain or body to alcohol itself. Unfortunately, few of these genes have explained, or have the potential to explain, the array of characteristics common among alcoholics, referred to as endophenotypes, which are antecedent to and also predict the development of alcoholism. For example, it is logical to presume that abnormalities in alcohol metabolism which increase the levels of acetalde-hyde (a toxin) in the bloodstream would reduce the likelihood that an individ-ual would drink to the point of becoming an alcoholic. But how would such a genetic trait also account for the association between the presence of attention deficit–hyperactivity disorder in childhood and the development of alcoholism as an adult? Are hyperactive youths less likely to be sickened by acetaldehyde? Unlikely. Are they more likely to drink in spite of the nausea? Perhaps.

In the quest to understand the genetic basis of alcoholism, it is not good enough simply to link individual genes to the occurrence of alcoholism. A true genetic characterization of *familial* alcoholism must also account for factors that are common among alcoholics—those evident before and after the development of the disease. We are certainly far from such a determin-ation. However, there is currently a strong movement within the USA to promote research that investigates the genetic underpinnings of these possible pre-existing characteristics (endophenotypes) which appear to predict the development of alcoholism.

12

Drinking 'rewards'

> ## Key points
>
> ◆ The neurotransmitter dopamine plays an important role in generating the feelings of pleasure that we perceive in response to alcohol as well as to food, sex, and other pleasurable stimuli.
>
> ◆ Excessive exposure to alcohol can alter brain systems in ways that diminish the brain's ability to perceive pleasure and cope with stress in the absence of alcohol.
>
> ◆ Alcohol stresses the body, activating the hypothalamic–pituitary–adrenocortical (HPA) axis which triggers the release of cortisol into the bloodstream. Chronic activation of the HPA axis can alter mood, disrupt the metabolism of sugars, and promote insomnia.
>
> ◆ Cumulative effects of depression, anxiety, and insomnia all contribute to the likelihood of relapse in abstinent alcoholics.

Why does an alcoholic drink? Why does anyone drink?

The answer to these questions seems obvious: it's because they like the way that alcohol makes them feel. Or they don't like the way that they feel without it. Still, it is difficult to understand why anyone would use alcohol to the point of sacrificing their homes, their jobs, their families, even their lives.

What makes an alcoholic crave alcohol so? Does drinking really make them feel that good? Or does alcohol just numb them to all of the bad that they feel (or both)? These are the types of questions that researchers have been stumbling over for years. They have spent decades studying the brains and behaviors of rats, mice, monkeys, pigeons, and humans. In the process, they have made some important advances that have shaped our understanding of the brain systems that are involved in the development of alcoholism as well as other addictions.

Pure pleasure

A key ingredient to the recipe of addictions appears to be a neurotransmitter molecule known as dopamine. Dopamine is produced by a small group of cells (neurons) in the middle of the brain called the substantia nigra and the ventral tegmental area (VTA). Dopamine released by these neurons is responsible for a variety of brain activities including learning, emotion, and bodily movements. It is the selective loss of these dopamine-containing neurons that causes the movement problems associated with Parkinson disease.

Dopamine is also an important part of the brain's so-called 'reward' or limbic system. This group of brain structures appears to be important for the perception of all things pleasurable to humans and animals: eating, sleeping, sex, drugs (and rock & roll).

All drugs of abuse, including alcohol, increase the levels of dopamine in the centers of the brain that signal pleasure. It is the positively reinforcing[1] actions at these brain sites which, at least initially, promote continued or excessive alcohol use. Over time, however, and in certain individuals, these systems can become deranged as the brain fights to restore biochemical normality. In some people, these systems may be impaired before alcohol is taken. These biochemical changes increase the amount of alcohol that is required to achieve the level of pleasure or sense of well-being that drinking normally produces. This encourages the individual to drink more and more.

Over time, animals forced to drink large amounts of alcohol have shown decreases in the levels of dopamine, serotonin, and other neurotransmitters in the brain that are involved with the regulation of mood and emotion. Decreases in the levels of these important neuromodulators are believed to have a negative effect on mood which worsens even more when the drinker abstains. Alcoholics who have developed a *dependence* on alcohol may experience serious symptoms of physical withdrawal in the absence of alcohol. While these symptoms provide a powerful motivation to drink in the short term, it is clear that physical withdrawal is only part of the addiction story. Negative mood states (depression) associated with alcohol withdrawal also create powerful cravings for alcohol and a preoccupation with drinking that may last well beyond any measurable physical symptoms of withdrawal.

Stress response

The relief of life stresses is another important motivation to drink alcohol for many people, and at low levels alcohol can provide a welcome respite from everyday worry which, at times, might even be beneficial. Unfortunately, chronic heavy drinking can lead to adaptations in the brain which ultimately increase sensitivity to stress, especially after alcohol is withdrawn. This can result in chronic anxiety and an impaired ability to cope with stressful life events without alcohol.

As discussed in Chapter 2, alcohol use has profound effects on the regulation of hormones within the brain. These effects include, among others, the disruption of a hormone system known as the hypothalamic–pituitary–adrenocortical (HPA) axis, which is the regulatory center for the body's response to stress. Alcohol acts as a stressor to the body, and even small amounts will activate the HPA axis, triggering the release of the stress hormone, cortisol, from the adrenal glands (near the kidneys) into the bloodstream. Cortisol release is the body's way of preparing for confrontation with danger. Cortisol's role in the metabolism of sugars, the regulation of blood pressure, and inflammatory and immune responses prepares the body for conflict and protects the body from injury. Increases in blood cortisol levels produce a heightened mental awareness and provide a quick burst of energy (via epinephrine release). Cortisol also decreases the perception of physical pain which permits a hasty retreat from danger even after sustaining an injury. These effects may be considered beneficial under certain circumstances; however, chronic activation of the HPA axis because of alcohol or other general life stressors can lead to a cascade of negative effects including impaired brain function, disrupted sugar metabolism, and decreased muscle and bone density.

Over time, the HPA axis appears to adjust its activity level to compensate for constant exposure to stress, leading to a reduction in blood cortisol levels in the absence of stress and an abnormal cortisol response to acute stress. Dysfunction of this system is believed to contribute to the development of anxiety and depressive mental disorders in addition to alcohol and substance abuse. Normal cortisol levels change according to circadian rhythms (sleep–wake cycle); therefore dysfunction of the HPA axis can also contribute to insomnia. This may be part of the reason why alcoholics often suffer from depression and anxiety disorders as well as insomnia, especially during periods of abstinence. Disruptions in the sleep–wake cycle of alcoholics can be severe and have been reported to persist after months or even years of abstinence. Accumulation of these stressors (depression, anxiety, insomnia, and physical withdrawal) in abstinent alcoholics is believed to contribute to the high rates of relapse observed in clinical treatment programs. In one study of alcoholic men, HPA responses reliably predicted relapse to drinking after 6 weeks of treatment.

The general activity of the HPA axis is determined by inherited as well as environmental factors. Mounting evidence suggests that some individuals may be biologically predisposed to abnormalities in HPA axis regulation prior to developing alcoholism. The specific brain systems involved in these regulatory processes are complex and involve brain reward centers including a system referred to as the 'extended amygdala'. The extended amygdala plays a crucial role in emotional behaviors and is able to over-ride the normal circadian regulation of the HPA axis. Abnormalities in the extended amygdala regulation of HPA function are believed to be another important contributor to the progression of alcoholism.

Motivation

An alcoholic rarely needs a 'reason' to drink. The activation of pleasure centers in the brain provides adequate motivation for most. Others seek only to escape the stresses of life for a time. Unfortunately, over time, the brain begins to resist the persistent activation of emotional centers, blunting emotional responses to pleasurable events, and increasing anxiety and mood disruption. This, in turn, drives a powerful craving for alcohol and fosters an increasing reliance upon alcohol to cope with the mounting stresses now associated with sobriety. As discussed in Chapter 9, individual vulnerability to the development of alcoholism appears to lie in a complex interaction between inherited, interpersonal, and environmental factors which ultimately dictate the responsiveness of brain reward centers as well as the activity of stress response systems.

13

Judgment and self-control

➲ Key points

- Many alcoholics possess behavioral traits and characteristics early in life that may directly or indirectly contribute to heavy drinking.

- Hyperactivity, impulsivity, aggression, and antisocial personality may lead to the disregard of social laws and norms as well as reckless alcohol use.

- These behavioral characteristics appear to reflect abnormalities in the frontal lobe of the brain, a region responsible for decision-making or so-called 'executive functions'.

It is worth noting that, drunk or sober, certain alcoholics tend to be trouble-makers. Whether he is the energetic life of the party or the town bully, this alcoholic usually gets noticed. More often than not, drunk or sober, the rationally minded will question his judgments. While there really is no such thing as an 'addictive personality', there are behavioral traits that are more commonly found among alcoholics even before they have had their first drink. Many of these—hyperactivity, impulsivity, aggressive and antisocial personalities—may also indirectly contribute to the development of alcoholism and drug abuse problems. Individuals who act impulsively or disregard social laws and norms are more likely to experiment with alcohol and drugs at an earlier age. They are also less likely to observe responsible drinking limits and habits once they begin to drink regularly. These individuals display impairments in judgment which may predispose them to escalate to alcoholic disease. Modern scientific advancements, particularly in brain imaging technology, have allowed scientists to home in on the specific brain systems which define the human sense of reason and judgment, judgments that we rely upon to regulate our actions appropriately. Deficiencies in these brain systems tend to run in alcoholic families and have been identified as risk factors for the development of alcoholism.

Loss of control model of alcoholism

Perhaps the greatest myth concerning the origins of alcoholism is the belief (held by many alcoholism researchers) that alcoholism actually begins with alcohol. While it is true that there is no such thing as a 'latent' alcoholic—you must drink alcohol to become an alcoholic—nevertheless, the disease of alcoholism cannot be explained *solely* by the actions of alcohol on the brain. It is not simply something that alcohol has *done to* the alcoholic or his brain. In fact, many alcoholics are struggling long before they begin to drink.

There are clear characteristic features found in many alcoholics that precede drinking which may directly or indirectly contribute to the development of alcoholism. These features include mental disorders and specific behavioral problems that may appear in childhood. As described in Chapter 10, alcoholism is sometimes associated with mental disorders which may lead to excessive drinking for 'self-medication' or simply the lack of better judgment. These psychiatric syndromes and personality characteristics contribute to a great deal of impairment and suffering in their own right. Studies have shown that alcoholics as a group are more likely to have been in trouble at school, had fights, been arrested, acquire a venereal disease, and to have been dishonorably discharged from the military *prior to* the development and diagnosis of alcoholism.

One area where such differences are particularly evident is in the regulation of natural drives and impulses. Many alcoholics have deficiencies in this area which can and do lead them into trouble, particularly during adolescence when drinking often begins.

Organized study of related mental conditions points to one specific area of the forebrain, known as the prefrontal cortex, as the command center for the regulation of behaviors. The prefrontal cortex is responsible for the integration of information from cognitive and emotional brain centers and the formulation of behavioral responses (referred to as executive functions). Dysfunction of this system can lead to acting on impulses without appropriately considering the consequences. Studies have found that abnormalities in the frontal lobe occur more often in children with large numbers of alcoholic relatives than in children with no alcoholic relatives. These abnormalities are associated with the development of behavioral problems such as attention deficit–hyperactivity disorder and conduct disorder, which are both strong predictors

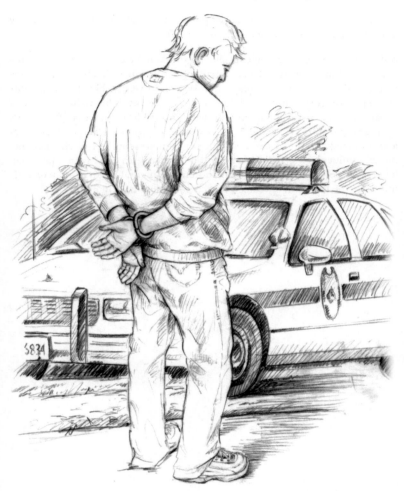

Figure 13.1 'Errors in judgment.' Artwork by Lorie Gavulic.

of alcoholism. Abnormalities in executive functions may result from inherited or environmental factors which influence brain development in childhood and adolescence. Chronic stress, poor nutrition, childhood trauma, or abuse can interfere with the normal development of these brain systems, leaving the individual lacking in important mental tools required to cope with the challenges of the adult world. Excessive drinking and drug use in adolescence can also dramatically affect the development of frontal brain systems and may lead to permanent impairments in executive functions.

Although these factors are not specific for drinking behaviors, they are important contributors to the development of alcohol use disorders, and they predict a disease course of greater duration and severity. This fact highlights the important role of healthy childhood development in the reduction of risk for alcoholism, especially in children with known developmental risk factors or a family history of alcoholism. Exposure to poverty, trauma, neglect, or abuse during childhood can result in permanent neurological changes that directly influence the skill set that will be available to cope with adult challenges. These increases in physical and environmental burdens may directly influence the risk of developing a drinking problem later in life.

Section 4

Treating alcoholism

Formula for longevity: Have a chronic disease and take care of it.

Oliver Wendell Holmes

14

Treating alcoholism

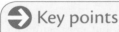 Key points

- There is no single approach to the treatment of alcoholism that has proven to be effective.

- Strategies for treatment tend to vary with the philosophy of the provider.

- Modern trends toward alcoholism treatment have moved away from lengthy and expensive inpatient care to community centers relying upon teams of mental health professionals.

Sometimes people recover from an illness without professional help. This is called spontaneous remission, 'spontaneous' meaning that the remission cannot be explained. Others prefer to call this phenomenon 'natural recovery' because the individual can usually give a reason why he decided to stop drinking or to stop drinking abusively. Spontaneous remission happens in almost every illness, including alcoholism. Before treatment can be judged to be effective, it must be shown to be superior to no treatment.

Usually studies comparing treated and untreated groups are needed in order to show effectiveness. However, some treatments are so effective that such comparative studies are not needed. Penicillin for pneumonia is an example. But it is a mistake to judge the effectiveness of a treatment by what happens to one, two, or a small group of patients. Even patients with terminal cancer sometimes recover 'spontaneously', and the history of medicine is a graveyard of treatments that were worthless but flourished because people tend to get over things anyhow.

There is no penicillin for alcoholism. Studies are needed. Some of the treatments discussed have never been studied; others have been studied, but not well. It may be a slight exaggeration, but only slight, to say that no study has proved beyond question that one treatment for alcoholism is superior to another treatment. Some studies argue that treatment has little long-term impact compared with no treatment at all.

Nevertheless, alcoholics seek help and people try to help them. Uncertainty about the results of treatment has not and should not discourage this effort.

Who is providing treatment? What treatments are available?

The tendency toward alcoholism may be inherited, but most authorities believe that alcoholism is partly learned (and thus psychological) and the learning takes place in a particular social environment—hence the term 'psychosocial'. Which is most important—heredity or learning—is not resolved, and the mix may differ in different people, but the issue is not purely academic. Treatment often depends on the treater's judgment about whether biological or psychosocial influences predominate.

Therapists who believe that alcoholism is mostly learned tend to believe that it can be unlearned. They believe that moderate drinking can be a proper goal of treatment. Those who minimize the role of learning tend to view alcoholism as an incurable condition for which total abstinence from alcohol is the only appropriate goal. Treatment philosophies differ in different parts of the USA and in different countries. In the USA, the total abstinence philosophy associated with AA is more common, although there are indications that this may be changing. The National Institute on Alcohol Abuse and Alcoholism has suggested that, for some alcoholics, a return to social drinking may be possible. In the UK, where AA is less influential, it is widely held that many alcoholics, particularly moderate alcoholics, can successfully 'return' to moderate drinking.

Sometimes the term 'biopsychosocial' is substituted for psychosocial, meaning that the therapist acknowledges that biological factors are important while continuing to maintain that psychological and social factors are equally important. This point of view has a certain face validity and is 'politically correct'. It pleases the biologists as well as the psychologists and sociologists—all toilers in the vineyards of alcoholism research and treatment. Hopefully, there is more to the 'multivariant' point of view than diplomacy. Each component of the biopsychosocial perspective is rooted in observation.

Alcoholism, for example, has been called a bad habit, and it certainly is, if bad habit means conditioned reflex. Conditioning involves semi-involuntary responses to stimuli or cues that trigger a need to drink. Conditioning is in the domain of psychology, even if mediated in the brain. However, if alcoholism is a bad habit, it is a bad habit that some people acquire more easily than others. It seems clear that people are 'born' with a susceptibility to certain bad habits and a resistance to others. Heredity seems to explain this variability more than any other influence.

As for psychosocial factors, presumably people drink for reasons, and the reasons may be psychological (a wish to feel happy) or social (a wish to feel less shy in groups). But psychological theorists do not rely merely on such commonplace examples. The 'learning model', as it is called, gains its strength from studies where people are given what they think is an alcoholic beverage. The subjects react as if they were drunk even when the experimenter cheats and doesn't put alcohol in the drinks. The more alcohol-dependent subjects are conditioned by long experience to react to drinking cues, and they react that way even when the vodka and tonic contains nothing but tonic. In other words, they *learned* to 'lose control' (believed by some to be the *sine qua non* of the 'disease model' of alcoholism) and they unlearn it with proper treatment. So the theory goes. Nobody denies the role of expectation in drinking behavior, but few believe that expectation alone causes a person to become alcoholic. However, some do, and the explanation goes as follows: the child of an alcoholic says to himself, 'Dad was alcoholic and therefore I'll become one', and he becomes one.

Not even the most ardent learning theorist believes that it is that simple. A shot of whiskey, downed straight, has effects that far exceed those based solely on expectation. You can fool an experimental subject when a small amount of alcohol is diluted in tonic water, but no one is fooled when a large amount of alcohol is added. There are biological responses to alcohol, if consumed in sufficient amounts, that cannot be explained by expectation or learning.

The social model emphasizes the importance of availability of alcohol, the effects of peer pressure, and the influence of cultural values, attitudes, and mores that regulate the use of alcohol. Alcoholism, in this model, is viewed as a 'social career' more or less like becoming an accountant or robber. Like the learning model, the importance of social factors cannot be denied. First, there must be alcohol for people to drink alcohol, and society usually provides it. In some Islamic countries possession of alcohol is a serious crime, even punishable by death. In these countries alcoholic beverages are effectively unavailable even though the ingredients for making alcohol—yeast, sugar, and water—are ubiquitous. Making alcohol very expensive is another possible way of limiting its availability. But studies show that in other countries where citizens are less passionately dedicated to drinking, increasing the price of alcohol does indeed reduce its consumption, at least among those who do not consume much anyway. There is no evidence that higher prices reduce drinking among the dependent drinkers we call alcoholic, nor is there any evidence that other social measures, such as closing down bars early or taking drastic action against drinking drivers, reduce drinking by the heaviest drinkers. Social pressure, more than anything else, may have contributed to the modest decline in consumption of alcohol, similar to the decline in cigarette smoking, as shared smoke has been shown to have deleterious effects on others.

It has been said that the three basic needs of mankind—food, security, and love—are so intertwined that is it difficult to tell whether a person is searching for one or the other. Thus it is hard to separate biological, psychological, and social factors in alcoholism. People who treat alcoholism generally acknowledge the multifactorial nature of the problem, while emphasizing an aspect most congruent with their training and beliefs.

The providers include social workers, psychologists, psychiatrists, other physicians, and alcoholism counselors, many of whom are recovered alcoholics.[1] Often treaters work together in a shared practice setting, and may function as a team managing different aspects of the patient's treatment and recovery.

Alcoholism is often ignored by physicians, and it is generally agreed that physicians are less active in treating the illness than they should be. Psychiatrists are often reluctant to see alcoholics, and when treating a patient with a drinking problem, some psychiatrists interpret the drinking as symptomatic of some other condition and ignore it.

Naturally, those who believe that alcoholism is *not* a disease do not expect doctors to help alcoholics and indeed would prefer that they do not try (except of course for medical complications, such as cirrhosis and delirium tremens). Some alcoholics reject any treatment that does not come from other alcoholics. 'How can anyone help an alcoholic who has not been one?' goes the reasoning. The same principle could apply to any condition. How can anyone treat cancer or diabetes who has not been diabetic or had cancer? Some feel that they can, and do, with some success.

Trends

A large number of reports in recent years have indicated that alcoholic patients benefit as much from brief outpatient services as they do from inpatient care. For more than two decades in the USA, treatment of alcoholism was concentrated at inpatient facilities modeled after the so-called Minnesota Plan. Patients were admitted for a period of several weeks and spent from early morning to late in the evening participating in group therapy, AA meetings, individual therapy, and educational activities, as well as a good deal of walking and performance of mild exercise. Sometimes patients spent time on the 'hot seat' where their faults were dissected with gusto by the other patients. The treatment philosophy was based on principles of AA, including the need for total abstinence.

The treatment was expensive, costing upwards of $25 000. As long as insurance companies ('third parties') picked up the bill, the system became increasingly popular, and even small cities would have at least one alcoholism and drug inpatient facility. Then insurers became aware of the lack of evidence supporting the effectiveness of long-term hospitalization and began curtailing reimbursements, encouraging brief outpatient therapies. Unfortunately, outpatient treatment is most effective only if the alcoholic is able to stop drinking long enough to participate, and this is often not likely for severely affected alcoholics. In the late 1990s, the American Society on Addiction Medicine developed guidelines for the use of inpatient versus outpatient treatment. These guidelines acknowledge the need for hospitalization if the alcoholic has complications of depression, or other psychiatric disorders, or during alcohol withdrawal has significant risk for seizures or delirium tremens. The guidelines have helped to modify restrictions on inpatient or residential treatment, while curtailing unnecessary use.

A similar trend away from lengthy hospitalization has occurred in the UK, where there has been increasing emphasis on community-based multidisciplinary teams. The teams are usually based in a building away from any hospital; they include psychiatric nurses, a psychologist, a social worker, counselors, and administrators/clerks. Some teams have a psychiatric consultant. The team members are involved in consultation, education, counseling and advisory services, and sometimes skills training. The staff size varies considerably, with as many as 50 members on some teams and as few as two to three on others.

In addition, there are several hundred day centers in the UK, mostly in inner cities. Most provide food and shelter and help with welfare rights and accommodation problems. A few offer individual counseling, group psychotherapy, drama therapy, and relaxation groups. Finally, there are residential hostel projects scattered throughout the UK. Most provide 12 or fewer beds plus day care.

Residential projects involve stays ranging from three months to a year or more. They attract problem drinkers who are homeless and those who are single, unemployed, and male. The goal is to permit people to spend time in an alcohol-free environment and learn to break their dependence on drinking.

Since the 1960s the National Health Service has supported treatment units (ATUs). Those that operate as separate units within hospitals are becoming almost obsolete, with patient care shifted to the community. Serious withdrawal symptoms are treated in a general or psychiatric hospital ward, although, as is true in the USA, home detoxification has become increasingly common.

15

Psychological approaches to the treatment of alcoholism

One thing about alcohol: it works. It may destroy a man's career, ruin his marriage, turn him into a zombie unconscious in a hall-way—but it works. On short term, it works much faster than a psychiatrist or a priest or the love of a husband or a wife. Those things ... they all take time. They must be developed ... But alcohol is always ready to go to work at once. Then minutes, half an hour, the little formless fears are gone or turned into harmless amusement. But they come back. Oh yes, and they bring re-enforcements.

Charles Orson Gorham

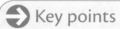 Key points

◆ Over the years, various behavioral and psychotherapeutic approaches have been applied to the treatment of alcoholism.

◆ Psychotherapy, in an individual or group setting, emphasizes the resolution of internal conflicts that may contribute to drinking problems.

◆ Behavioral therapy attempts to over-ride conditioned associations between drinking and any positive feelings or sensations that alcohol may produce.

◆ Cognitive therapy seeks to reduce alcohol use by changing the alcoholic's attitudes and beliefs concerning drinking.

The following chapters provide a review of what is availalbe to help the alcoholic. The discussion encompasses both psychological and medical domains, with most of the medical approaches developing in recent years. The present chapter highlights the multitude of psychological methods that have been drawn upon for the treatment of alcoholism over the past century. The majority of these procedures are based upon very early psychological theories, and their use, in general, has waxed and waned over time depending upon changing trends in the field and their particular popularity. Although the discussion may be *waxing nostalgia* for the expert, many of these approaches are still widely used today and warrant comment of their effectiveness. The discussion tends to be critical, but there is no choice if you respect evidence. Alcoholics Anonymous, some say the best treatment of all, is discussed in Chapter 17.

Psychotherapy

There are several schools of psychotherapy, but they have one thing in common: they involve two or more persons talking to each other, one of whom is the psychotherapist, a trained expert in the treatment being offered. It is important to distinguish psychotherapy from counseling. As a rule, psychotherapy costs more than counseling, takes longer, and is usually performed by qualified psychotherapists, psychiatrists, or psychologists trained in a particular method of psychotherapy.

Psychotherapy may be individual or take place in a group. In the group setting, as in the individual, it is important to distinguish between educational and supportive groups, and specialized group therapy which is given by qualified individuals trained in a specific therapeutic approach. In some instances, individual and group psychotherapy are combined in an integrated program.

To show that a particular treatment is useful, three questions must be asked.

◆ Would the patient have recovered without any treatment?

◆ Would he have done as well or better with another treatment?

◆ Is his improvement related to non-specific aspects of a treatment?

'Non-specific aspects' include, in Peter Medawar's words, the 'assurance of a regular sympathetic hearing, the feeling that somebody is taking his condition seriously, the discovery that others are in the same predicament, the comfort of learning that his condition is explicable (which does not depend on the explanation being the right one)'. These factors are common to most forms of psychological treatment, and the good they do cannot be credited to any one treatment in particular.

Behavior therapy

There are two kinds of behavior therapy with two different ancestries. One comes from Pavlov, who conditioned dogs. The other comes from B.F. Skinner, who conditioned pigeons. Behavior therapy, in other words, is conditioning therapy by another name.

Pavlov found that if dogs repeatedly heard a bell before eating, eventually bells alone would make them salivate. And if you shocked the dog's foot every time he heard a bell, he would soon respond to bells in the same way he did to shock—by withdrawing the foot.

For many years attempts have been made to condition alcoholics to dislike alcohol. Alcoholics are asked to taste or smell alcohol just before a pre-administered drug makes them nauseated. Repeated pairing of alcohol and nausea results in a conditioned response—after a while alcohol alone makes them nauseated. Thereafter, it is hoped, the smell or taste of alcohol will cause nausea and discourage drinking.

Instead of pairing alcohol with nausea, other therapists have associated it with pain, shocking patients just after they drink, or with the panic experienced from not being able to breathe by giving them a drug that causes very brief respiratory paralysis. Others have trained patients to imagine unpleasant effects from drinking, hoping to set up a conditioned response without causing so much actual distress.

Does it work? Some degree of conditioning is usually established, but it is uncertain how long the conditioning lasts. The largest study that involved con-ditioning alcoholics was conducted several decades ago in Seattle, Washington. More than 4000 patients conditioned to feel nauseated when exposed to alcohol were studied 10–15 years after treatment. Half were abstinent, which is an impressive recovery rate compared with other treatments. The patients who did best had booster sessions, i.e. they came back to the clinic after the initial treatment to repeat the conditioning procedure. Of those who had booster sessions, 90 percent were abstinent. Based on this study, the nausea treatment for alcoholism would seem to be an outstanding success. Why hasn't it been universally accepted?

One reason is that the results can be attributed to factors other than condi-tioning. The patients in the study were a special group. Generally they were well educated, had jobs, and were well off financially. They may not have received the treatment otherwise, since the clinic where they were treated is private and costs money. Indeed, the patients who did best, it turned out, had the most money. Studies of alcoholics have often shown that certain subject characteristics are more predictive of successful treatment outcome than the type of treatment administered. These include job stability, living with a relative, absence of a criminal record, and living in a rural community. In the Seattle study there was no control group which did not receive conditioning therapy. It is possible that the select group of patients, many having characteristics that favor a good outcome, would have done as well without conditioning.

Furthermore, in conditioning treatments, motivation is important. Treatment is voluntary and involves acute physical discomfort, so presumably few would consent to undergo the therapy who were not strongly motivated to stop drinking. The Seattle study makes this point graphically clear. Those who came back for booster sessions did better than those who did not, but another group did better still—those who wanted to come back but could not because they lived too far from the hospital. All of these people remained abstinent.

In 1991 the first study comparing aversion therapy with treatment that did not include aversion therapy was published. The results were similar to those reported above. The 'controls' were listed in a national registry—perhaps not the ideal controls. However, the two groups were matched on such variables as income, and the study provided further evidence that aversion helps selected individuals.

Other studies of the Pavlovian type of therapy for alcoholism (including chemical, electrical, and verbal conditioning) have been less ambitious and the results have been mixed. To the extent that they seem to help, success may be attributable to factors unrelated to conditioning, such as patient selection, patient cooperation, and so on. Another factor may also promote at least short-term success. It is called the Hawthorne effect and refers to the enthusiasm that therapists often have for any treatment that is new. The enthusiasm may be infectious, and patients who are enthusiastic themselves about a particular treatment may do somewhat better, for a time, than those who are neutral or unenthusiastic.

The same considerations apply to therapy based on the work of B.F. Skinner, which is called operant conditioning. There is a large scientific literature based on this work, but the basic ideas are simple. People behave like pigeons in the sense that they do things which are rewarded and avoid doing things which are punished. This has led to a type of treatment known as token economy. Anything a patient does that is believed to be good for him is rewarded (often literally with tokens which are exchangeable for food, money, and other desirable things). Anything he does that is bad for him is punished (usually simply by withholding the reward). In this manner an attempt is made to 'shape' the behavior of patients in directions that are beneficial to them, with the hope that the new behavior—abstinence or controlled drinking—will permanently replace the less beneficial kind.

Does this actually happen? Most treatments of this kind take place in institutional settings, and whether the new behavior brought about in the institution 'sticks' in the outside world is not known.

One final word needs to be said about conditioning therapies. Alcoholics, by the time they seek professional help, have already suffered bitterly from their drinking, but this has not deterred them from continuing to drink. Being made to vomit or having their hand shocked by a friendly therapist is incomparably less excruciating than the physical and mental anguish that alcoholics normally experience: the morning heaves, the shakes, the crushing weight of conscience. There is a sizable delay, to be sure, between the drinking and the anguish, and for conditioning in the literal sense to occur the delay should be shorter. But the effects of heavy drinking are so punishing that one would expect some kind of deterrent effect. After all, some people become sick after eating a pork chop and thereafter avoid pork chops. The need to drink must be compelling indeed, given the infinitely greater misery that comes from drinking. This is what addiction really means, as was movingly described by William James (who had a brother who was alcoholic):

> The craving for a drink in real dipsomaniacs [drunkards] is of a strength of which a normal person can form no conception. Were a keg of rum in one corner of a room and were a cannon constantly discharging balls between me and it, I could not refrain from passing before that cannon in order to get the rum. If a bottle of brandy stood at one hand and the pit of hell yawned at the other, and I were convinced that I should be pushed in as sure as I took one glass, I could not refrain.

James then gives two case-histories:

> A few years ago a tippler was put in an almshouse. Within a few days he had devised various expedients to procure rum, but failed. At length, however, he hit upon one which was successful. He went into the wood yard of the establishment, placed one hand upon the block, and with an axe in the other, struck it off at a single blow. With the stump raised and streaming he ran into the house and cried, 'Get me some rum! My hand is off!' In the confusion and bustle of the occasion a bowl of rum was brought, into which he plunged the bleeding

member of his body, then raising the bowl to his mouth, drank freely, and exultantly exclaimed, 'Now I am satisfied.' [There also was the] man who, while under treatment for inebriety, during four weeks secretly drank the alcohol from six jars containing morbid specimens. On asking him why he had committed this loathsome act, he replied: 'Sir, it is as impossible for me to control this diseased appetite as it is for me to control the pulsations of my heart'.

To control 'this diseased appetite' with a few sessions of conditioning therapy seems a little like attacking an elephant with a peashooter. However, one thing can be said in favor of conditioning therapy: it is inexpensive, probably does no harm, and arises from a scientific tradition that emphasized evidence more than faith.

Cognitive therapies

'Cognitive' means to learn or know. In recent years, several new 'cognitive' approaches to the treatment of alcoholism have been proposed. They are called by a variety of names but have two elements in common: they are brief, and they involve trying to change a patient's way of thinking.

The 'disease' model compares the alcoholic with a rider who may believe that he can control his horse, but this is an illusion. The horse is the master. All the rider can do is get off—give up alcohol. Not so, says the cognitive therapist. The patient can guide the horse. He can change his drinking behavior by changing his thoughts. Here are some approaches to thought management and the names that they go by.

Cognitive-behavior therapy has a general goal and specific technique for controlling harmful drinking. The word behavior simply refers to the way people behave—not conditioning. Looking for a better treatment for depression, the American psychiatrist Aaron Beck found that depressed people stopped being depressed if they stopped having depressing thoughts. Although this sounds easier said than done, he insisted that depressed patients did not have to have depressed thoughts and that he could help them to have undepressed thoughts. He developed a rather simple set of techniques for doing this, and cognitive therapy became widely popular for almost every known psychiatric condition, including alcoholism.

In the case of depression, studies show that cognitive therapy is sometimes as good as drugs and that a combination of cognitive therapy and drugs sometimes produces the best results of all. Evidence that it is effective for the addictions, including alcoholism, has been mixed, with some studies showing that it helps and others showing that it does not. In any case, cognitive therapy for alcoholism, going under several names, has been the most studied of all alcoholism treatments and has the advantage of being brief and therefore cost-effective. Long and expensive inpatient programs for alcoholics (often following the Minnesota Plan) have been shown in many studies to be no more effective than brief and relatively inexpensive outpatient treatment. The latter usually consists of giving advice and sometimes performing cognitive therapy, as well as encouraging the patient to attend Alcoholics Anonymous, at least in the USA.

Cognitive therapy aimed at changing a person's behavior (which is why it is called cognitive-behavior therapy) often begins with attempts to help the patient identify thought patterns that undermine self-esteem and engender anxiety. The therapist teaches the patient how to identify negative assumptions that the patient makes about self and others, and suggests ways to reframe problems and behaviors more realistically. To some extent this is based on the assumption that people cannot have two opposing thoughts simultaneously. One cannot think, 'I am miserable and therefore must drink' and simultaneously think 'I'm feeling pretty good, so why should I drink?' Instead the person should say, 'I am a unique individual. Just because I am the son of my father does not mean I should behave like my father'. The therapist points out 'errors of logic' that the patient can correct if he perceives the errors to be errors and practices thinking good thoughts about himself. The practice takes the form of self-statements, another way of saying that the patient must learn to talk to himself. He should avoid talking to himself out loud in public—those around might misunderstand—but by suspending the use of his vocal cords a person can carry on a conversation with himself without seeming psychotic. In privacy, speaking one's own thoughts aloud can sometimes reveal errors in thinking, similar to trying to explain a thought to another person. Verbalizing a thought often exposes unrecognized assumptions that may be inaccurate.

After several sessions with a cognitive therapist the patient has usually acquired a collection of self-statements, sometimes called 'bumper stickers'. Common ones include, 'There is only today' and 'All of us will be dead in 100 years'. (The latter sounds depressing but actually can be reassuring if the person worries overly about how others view him.) A favorite bumper sticker comes from William James: 'Wisdom is about learning what to overlook'. This covers a whole range of irritations at home, at work, and driving in heavy traffic.

These are self-statements intended to help patients think better of themselves (and probably, by extension, think better of others). Presumably, it would help anybody who 'automatically' reacts negatively to everything and everybody around them, often including the therapist. Thinking, it turns out, need not be entirely automatic. The thinker need not be entirely a passive victim of his thoughts. Patients are sometimes amazed to learn how easily they can substitute constructive healthy thoughts for gloomy thoughts. Probably some people possess the skill more than others (maybe because of genes), and, like all arts, the art of positive thinking requires effort and concentration. The experienced cognitive therapist can help even those congenital 'awfulizers' from interpreting whatever happens to them as awful.

Cognitive therapy is more active than many talk therapies because it requires that the alcoholic learn and rehearse new responses to new thinking patterns, identify and practice different coping behaviors, learn new social skills and apply those skills in sessions, learn how to monitor moods and respond to unanticipated mood changes, and plan and implement lifestyle changes. It is not enough to talk about feelings; the alcoholic must practice the new behavior until the behavior becomes comfortable. One form of cognitive-behavior therapy called 'dialectical behavior therapy' emphasizes learning new skills of interpreting other people's behavior, deciding how to respond, and developing specific scripts and scenarios

One reason alcoholics feel hopeless about their drinking is that they painfully remember all the times they managed to abstain entirely or moderate their intake only to go back to heavy drinking. The serious form of alcohol dependence called alcoholism is, by most definitions, a chronic condition characterized by frequent relapse. *Relapse prevention* is a name for one form of cognitive therapy. It involves identifying 'high-risk' situations associated with relapse. This may differ from drinker to drinker, but common high-risk situations include parties, celebrations, holiday, hunger, fatigue, and loneliness. When situations most likely to produce relapse are identified in a particular patient, coping skills are then imparted for dealing with the situations. This may involve avoiding parties or, on the contrary, learning new social skills so the person can feel comfortable at the party while nursing an orange juice.

Some therapists believe that this can be achieved by a sheer act of will. Others disagree and point out that many aspects of a person's social life may not be manipulable in the office of a therapist and may be crucial in determining whether the person relapses. These critics view alcohol consumption as a social behavior driven by social forces. Relapse is believed to represent a response to social pressures such as unemployment, marital conflict, social isolation, and peer influence. The changes that the patient needs in order to avoid relapse do not occur entirely within the person. The therapist should help find him a job, conduct marriage counseling, and help him find a friend or hobby. This may involve increasing the drinker's job-finding skills, or getting him a driver's license, and taking out a newspaper subscription. This is sometimes called community reinforcement. It requires a lot of time and effort on the part of the therapist, more than most therapists are able to provide even if inclined to do so.

Practitioners of relapse prevention do not always strive to keep the patient (or client as he is often called) from drinking entirely. Moderation may be the goal, particularly for patients with mild forms of alcohol dependence. Of course, relapse prevention in the severely alcoholic person is more difficult to achieve, and most agree that much depends on whether the alcoholic is 'prepared' to stop drinking. This is based on the observation that people seem to stop drinking when they are ready to do so, and if they are not ready then professional intervention is of little help.

Carlo DiClemente and William Miller, psychologists who have studied psychotherapy for alcoholics for many years, have proposed that when therapy is not useful, it may be that the therapist needs to see the problem from the same perspective as the alcoholic. In this way of thinking, behavior change occurs in evolving stages, and motivation to change is dependent on the stage the alcoholic has reached. For example, if the alcoholic is beginning to think about getting sober because he was convicted of driving under the influence, the therapist might focus on how treatment and sobriety could influence legal consequences. The therapist's job is to identify the motivational factors for the alcoholic, and direct the therapy so that the alcoholic can use that motivation to reach his goals. It is usually evident that drinking is blocking ways of reaching goals, and sometimes the alcoholic can forgo drinking because the motivation to reach another goal is sufficiently strong and the goal appears feasible.

Cognitive-behavioral therapy goes by many names: CBT, relapse prevention training, social skills training, behavior self-control training, stress management, and others. They can all be given as individual therapy or in groups, and all involve changing a person's way of thinking. They have the advantage of being cost-effective, and have a more substantial database supporting reduction of alcoholic drinking and improving some aspects of quality of life.

Psychodynamic therapy

A historical method of psychotherapy is called psychodynamic therapy, and derives from the doctrines of Freud and his contemporaries, known as psychoanalysts. In psychodynamic theory, mental illness is attributed to unconscious conflicts that originate in infancy and early childhood. Because everyone has experienced psychological conflicts, the idea that mental illness arises from conflict remains speculative. Because drinking alcohol is an oral activity, alcoholism is thought to be related to conflicts involving feeding. Others hold that alcoholism is a form of self-destruction (which it obviously is) and has the same roots as depression. People have angry feelings toward others, cannot express them, and therefore become angry with themselves. Self-hatred is subjectively experienced as depression or leads to self-destructive acts such as alcoholism. Therapy consists of helping a person to recognize his unconscious drives and motives, which theoretically results in a happier and more mature person who does not drink as much.

Contemporary psychodynamic psychotherapies for addiction tend to emphasize the role of conflict and stress, poor self-esteem, inadequate emotional regulation, and difficulties in developing and maintaining satisfying relationships. Alcoholics often talk about feelings of rage, anxiety, depression, loneliness, emptiness, etc., which can be temporarily suppressed with alcohol, resulting in the idea that alcohol is being used to treat these feelings. This is called the 'self-medication hypothesis'. In this approach, alcoholics recognize and learn other ways of managing these feelings and are then able to stop using alcohol. Although this approach is intuitively attractive and seems logical, it has not been shown to be effective, perhaps because being in psychotherapy requires having strong feelings, which is what prompted drinking in the first place.

Another form of psychotherapy is based on the theories of Eric Berne and is called transactional analysis (TA). Dr Berne's ideas had much in common with those of Freud. Instead of id, ego, and superego, he substitutes the terms child, adult, and parent. These three *dramatis personae* of mental life are constantly feuding, just as members of a family quarrel, and the quarrels sometimes take the form of abnormal behavior. All people play games and 'sick' people play games calculated to make them losers. The alcoholic punishes other people by punishing himself and is the loser in the end. TA makes alcoholics aware of the games they play and encourages them to find other games that are less destructive. TA lends itself somewhat more to group therapy than does psychoanalysis or psychodynamic psychotherapy.

Summary

How effective is treatment? This question, often asked by patients, families, insurers, and managed care companies, was addressed by the Institute of Medicine (IOM) and reported to the public in 1990. The IOM concluded that a better question would be 'Which kinds of individuals, with what kinds of alcohol problems, are likely to respond to what kinds of treatments by achieving which kinds of goals when delivered by which kinds of practitioners?' Heterogeneity is inherent in the treatment field, and comparison of treatment methods across studies is complex and challenging. Nevertheless, Emrick in 1974 and Miller in 2000 reported that, using data from published well-designed and controlled studies, the outcome generally fell into the range of one-third abstinent, one-third with marked improvement, and one-third unchanged in drinking behavior. This outcome is probably analogous to that for treated hypertension, diabetes, and other chronic diseases with individual variability in disease course and treatment response.

16

Medications to treat the alcoholic

> **Key points**
>
> ◆ A wide variety of medications are now available to aid in the recovery from alcoholism.
>
> ◆ Medications developed to reduce alcohol use act through a variety of mechanisms. Newer therapies attempt to address the underlying neurobiological processes associated with relapse.
>
> ◆ Other medications offer relief from the distress associated with alcohol withdrawal and abstinence.

Medication to reduce alcohol use

In Sears Roebuck mail order catalogs in the early 1900s two pages were devoted to medication therapies for morphine addiction and alcoholism. The medication being sold for morphine addiction consisted mainly of alcohol; a good part of the medication for alcoholism consisted of a tincture of opium, a relative of morphine. Whether morphine addicts became alcoholics as a result of the treatment, or vice versa, is not known, but it illustrates the long history of giving a medication that affects mood and behavior to relieve the effects of another drug that affects mood and behavior. Substitution therapy reached a pinnacle with the widespread, officially sanctioned, and clinically useful substitution of methadone (an addicting substance like heroin) for heroin. Heroin itself was introduced at the turn of the century as a 'heroic' cure for morphine addiction and was also believed to be useful for alcoholism.

Historically some Alcoholics Anonymous (AA) members, and some alcoholism treatment professionals, have argued that alcoholics should not take any medications. At one extreme, alcoholics have been told that even aspirin and Tylenol® should be avoided, although the AA Big Book states that alcoholics should take medication as prescribed by a physician. Prior to the emergence of studies documenting that alcoholics often have comorbid psychiatric disorders, many AA groups criticized use of antidepressants and mood stabilizers, believing that these medications 'are mood-altering drugs and dangerous for alcoholics'. (Some still hold that belief.) Many alcoholics now receive treatment for comorbid psychiatric disorders (see Chapter 10) and medication is more readily accepted.

Antidepressants, anxiolytics, and mood stabilizers

Medications widely prescribed to alcoholics mainly consist of medications for anxiety and depression. Antidepressants are more often prescribed than anti-anxiety medications such as Valium®, Xanax®, and others in a class called benzodiazepines, more often called just 'benzos.' The latter medications have some effects similar to those of alcohol (they calm and relax) and are useful in relieving the jitteriness that follows heavy drinking, so that they may be useful in stopping a drinking bout. Whether they stop the resumption of drinking—the test of a medication's true worth in treating alcoholism—is debatable, and many clinicians feel that they do not.

Benzodiazepines are sometimes used in excess by alcoholics, and sometimes in combination with alcohol. This may not be as harmful as it sounds since they have a low range of toxicity, but some people can become addicted in the literal sense of needing increasingly larger amounts and having serious withdrawal symptoms when they stop taking them. These medications have contributed little to the management of alcoholism, and some clinicians feel strongly that they should not be given to alcoholics for extended periods.

Antidepressant medications are useful to treat depression in alcoholics, and appear to be effective when alcoholics become seriously depressed (which is common). However, when antidepressants have been studied to decrease alcohol abuse, they seem to have only a modest impact. The group of antidepressant medications that enhance the effects of the neurotransmitter serotonin on brain cells, called selective serotonin reuptake inhibitors (SSRIs), are most often used because they have more tolerable side effects and less risk if taken in overdose. Some of these medications (citalopram, nefazadone, sertraline, and fluoxetine) reduce drinking in animals and humans.

Fluoxetine also had mixed effects on abstinence in some studies. When the alcoholics in these studies were grouped into different types of alcoholism, fluoxetine and sertraline appeared to have a differential effect on drinking.

Alcoholics with no family history of alcoholism, compared with those with close relatives who were alcoholic, had a better initial response and longer duration of response to these medications. Whether this might be true for other SSRIs needs to be studied. The results are preliminary and need to be confirmed, yet may be of some help in choosing an antidepressant. Some of the older antidepressants, called tricyclic antidepressants (TCAs), were successful in reducing concurrent alcohol use when given to alcoholics for depression. TCAs have more side effects and can be lethal in overdose; thus they are not widely used despite the positive reports.

Lithium, a drug useful in the treatment of mania, has been given to alcoholics, and early reports indicated that some people have benefited from it. Since early reports often indicate that a particular treatment is useful, only to be refuted by later reports, lithium therapy was viewed with both interest and skepticism. The skepticism was reinforced when a large multihospital study in the USA failed to find that lithium was useful for alcoholism. Many people with manic-depressive disorder, now called bipolar disorder, are alcoholic and often drink more when they are manic than when they are depressed. Therefore, for these people, using lithium to help reduce manic episodes may result in reduced alcoholic drinking.

From a theoretical viewpoint, it is interesting that antianxiety drugs and most antidepressant drugs do not seem to deter alcoholics from using alcohol. If alcoholics drink because they feel anxious and depressed, one would assume that relieving the anxiety and depression would reduce interest in alcohol more than these drugs seem to do. Other treatments that have been tried are LSD and large doses of vitamins, with no convincing evidence that they help.

Aversive therapy

A medication commonly prescribed for alcoholism over the past 25 years is one that has no effect on anxiety or depression or apparently anything else unless combined with alcohol. This, of course, is Antabuse®.

This drug makes people physically ill when they drink. When it was first used in the early 1950s, Antabuse® got a bad name for two reasons. First, like most highly touted treatments, it was not the panacea that enthusiastic supporters had hoped it would be. Secondly, some people taking the drug died after drinking. It was later learned that the drug could be given in smaller amounts and still produce an unpleasant reaction when combined with alcohol, but death was exceedingly rare.

127

Partly because of the bad reputation it obtained in the early years, it has per-haps been underused since then. The more dogmatic members of AA view Antabuse® as somehow incompatible with the spirit of AA, and many alcohol-ics resist taking the drug on the grounds that it is a 'crutch'.

Antabuse® has not been entirely popular with doctors for another reason. Some still believe they must give an Antabuse® 'challenge' test before pre-scribing the drug for indefinite periods. This test consists of giving the patient Antabuse® for a few days and then giving them a small amount of alcohol to demonstrate what an Antabuse® reaction is like. The Antabuse® challenge test is no longer considered necessary or even desirable. Patients can be told what the effects of Antabuse® will be and this will have the same effect. One awk-ward aspect of the challenge test is that some patients have no reaction when given the alcohol, simply because people react very differently to both alcohol and Antabuse®, and the cautious doses of alcohol administered are too small to produce an effect.

However, the main problem with Antabuse® is not that patients drink after taking the drug, but that they stop taking the drug because they 'forget' to take it, or convince themselves that it is no longer necessary, or that there are sig-nificant side effects, or a myriad of rationalizations to stop taking it. Of course, this is true for drugs other than Antabuse®, and is true for the treat-ment of other diseases as well. Compliance is generally a major issue in medi-cine. Adapting to the reality that something is truly wrong with one's body, or mind, is a process that can take months or years, and taking medication con-sistently is a hard-learned skill.

In the first edition of *Alcoholism: the facts*, Don Goodwin proposed a strategy to be used with alcoholics starting Antabuse® which is given at the end of this chapter. The techniques to build rapport, develop self-confidence, and teach problem-solving that are described for use with Antabuse® can also be applied when the alcoholic is prescribed other medications, either for alcoholism or for associated mood or anxiety disorders.

Naltrexone

At the time of writing, two other medications have been approved by the US Food and Drugs Administration (FDA) to reduce alcohol craving. The first is naltrexone, which is marketed as Revia® in a tablet, and is also available as a monthly injection. Naltrexone works in the brain to block the same site that is activated by heroin and prescription pain medications, which are called opioids. This site, called the μ-receptor, is an important component of the brain's reward system. The μ-receptor may be involved in both the euphoria and craving for alcohol, opioids, and perhaps other substances, and some behaviors such as gambling. When the μ-receptor is blocked by naltrexone, it appears that the rewarding effect of alcohol in the brain is reduced. Some alcoholics report that naltrexone makes it possible to 'not think' about alcohol and therefore reduces the struggle to avoid drinking. It is possible that naltrexone may also reduce alcohol craving by reducing the brain's perception of the positive effects of alcohol.

There have been more than a dozen studies of naltrexone for alcoholism, of which the majority support reduction of drinking, if not total abstinence. It is important to note that, along with providing naltrexone, these research studies also provided some form of psychosocial treatment, usually cognitive-behavioral therapy (Chapter 15). The intensity of psychosocial treatment may be a factor in whether subjects were able to reduce alcohol use, but this is an ongoing research question. When compared with placebo, naltrexone plus psychosocial treatment extended the number of non-drinking days. Not all studies have shown benefits for this combination, but these studies were typically conducted in severe alcoholics with few support resources.

Naltrexone has fewer side effects than Antabuse® but may still cause nausea and may injure the liver. Since the liver is already at risk for many alcoholics, this side effect needs monitoring. Naltrexone may also cause headache, fatigue, lethargy, and dysphoria in some individuals. (Of course, continued alcohol use is likely to produce even more health problems for most people.) People who need opioid pain medication cannot take naltrexone because it blocks the pain reduction effects of these medications.

Naltrexone is now available in a monthly injection which was developed to help alcoholics improve compliance with the medication, as most people seem to forget to take the pill after a month or two. The injection is very expensive and not covered by many insurance companies in the USA. Perhaps the cost is why it has not been used widely despite the advantage of compliance.

Acamprosate

A second medication developed to reduce alcohol use, acamprosate, which is marketed as Campral®, was recently approved by the FDA. This medication has been available in Europe for more than 10 years, and there are extensive research studies supporting its effectiveness there. In the USA, acamprosate has been available for only a few years and not as many research studies have been reported.

The manner in which acamprosate works is not fully understood. It appears to restore balance in two of the major brain systems, the glutamate and GABA systems, although other neurotransmitter systems may be involved. These brain systems are strongly affected by alcohol, and are thought to produce many of the severe symptoms seen in alcohol withdrawal. Acamprosate seems to work best for alcoholics who have completed detox, and may work better for relapse prevention than treatment. Alcoholics appear to remain abstinent longer when taking acamprosate, and some report that preoccupation with alcohol is reduced or eliminated, without specific effects on mood or thinking.

Acamprosate has some adverse side effects, primarily nausea. Also, because it must be taken three times daily, many people have difficulty in remaining fully compliant. It is unknown whether acamprosate works when taken less regularly than recommended. Acamprosate does not interact with other medications and is not metabolized by the liver; thus it may be easily combined with medications prescribed for the variety of psychiatric and medical conditions commonly experienced by alcoholics.

As it appears that naltrexone and acamprosate work on different aspects of brain neurotransmitter function, would there be any advantage in combining them (other than the advantage to pharmaceutical companies)? There are conflicting reports about the effectiveness of using both medications together. A large and complicated research study was recently completed that specifically addressed this question. The study, sponsored by the National Institute on Alcohol Abuse and Alcoholism (NIAAA), was appropriately titled COMBINE. The design compared naltrexone alone with acamprosate alone and both of these drugs with naltrexone and acamprosate given together. The study also included a comparison of two different talk therapies, cognitive-behavioral therapy (CBT) and medical management. A total of 1383 subjects took one of the two medications, or the two medications combined, or placebo, for 16 weeks. Each subject was also enroled in either CBT or medication management, except for a group of 157 subjects who received only CBT. Subjects who received medication management came to the physician's office every two weeks for 30 minutes. Some visits were to talk about the medication and receive encouragement from staff, and others involved medical examinations and testing. CBT was given weekly and allowed for additional sessions if needed (up to 20). The results support the efficacy of naltrexone, whether given with CBT or with medical management, to reduce craving and enhance abstinence. The outcome for acamprosate was surprising—it was no better than placebo. This result is quite different from the majority of previous studies, and may require replication before concluding that acamprosate is not effective. Also, combining naltrexone with acamprosate did not have any advantage over naltrexone alone.

One interesting finding was that medical management was as effective as CBT when combined with naltrexone. This means that family practice doctors (and also other specialties) can give naltrexone, combined with periodic visits to the office, to treat alcoholism when specific psychotherapy or specialized treatment programs are not available. The medical management treatment program has been published by the NIAAA, and is available to the public. Obviously, some alcoholics have psychiatric disorders that need different treatment and complicate the course of recovery. These patients are best referred to mental health professionals.

Topiramate

Although there are no other medications approved by the FDA for alcoholism, there is growing evidence that a newer anticonvulsant called topiramate (trade name Topamax®) also reduces craving and extends time to relapse. Topiramate works on brain GABA and N-methyl-D-aspartate (NMDA) neurotransmitter systems, and may have some activity in reducing anxiety. As discussed in Chapter 12, anxiety is a frequent problem for alcoholics and is believed to contribute to alcohol cravings and relapse. Topiramate is best tolerated if it is begun at a low dose and gradually tapered to the therapeutic dose, taking several weeks to become effective. It tends to have unusual side effects including slowed cognition, word-finding difficulty, poor concentration, odd sensory feelings in extremities, called paresthesias, and weight loss. Nevertheless, two well-designed placebo-controlled studies have shown it to be effective in men with relatively severe alcoholism. Some other anticonvulsants (divalproex sodium and carbamazepine) have also been studied briefly with good response, suggesting that this group of medications may have some utility.

Treating comorbidity

The recognition of comorbid psychiatric disorders among alcoholics, and need for medication management, has prompted numerous questions from patients and their doctors. How does the physician know when medication might be helpful to the alcoholic? When should medications be prescribed? If the alcoholic is still drinking, how can one know which symptoms are from alcohol and which from depression? If he stops drinking will the depression symptoms go away? Should the medication be delayed until the alcoholic is sober for a period of time? If so, for how long? If the alcoholic relapses and is drinking, should he continue the medication? How does one know if the medication is working? What are the target symptoms? How long should the medication be continued?

Historically, alcoholic patients were admitted to an inpatient program, detoxed, and continued in treatment for several weeks. This provided a good opportunity to evaluate persistent symptoms and decide if the diagnosis of depression or anxiety was warranted. With the reduction in inpatient and residential treatment, the physician must now work with the family and/or support system, with the inherent inaccuracies. Many alcoholics continue to have low levels of insomnia, irritability, anxiety, depression, and fluctuating mood states for months into abstinence. Although minor compared with the stress of clinical depression, these symptoms produce daily discomfort and contribute to the difficulties of maintaining abstinence. There is no research to indicate whether treating these symptoms improves abstinence, but it seems likely that more humane management of distress would be useful. This syndrome has been called the 'post-acute withdrawal syndrome' or PAWS for short.

Nunes and Levin published a review of the current literature, including eight well-designed and carefully controlled studies of medication treatment for alcoholics with depression symptoms. They concluded that subjects seemed to respond better to antidepressants if they had been diagnosed and started on the medication at least a week after completing detox. There did not appear to be much difference between subjects who started medication as inpatients and subjects in an outpatient program. Of course, it is sometimes not possible for alcoholics with persistent depression to remain abstinent for several weeks after detox, and treatment in a residential program for three or four weeks may be necessary to prevent relapse before the antidepressant has developed an effect on symptoms. These studies supported the need for concurrent psychosocial treatment, as the antidepressant medication helped with depression symptoms but appeared to have little effect on continued drinking. There are virtually no data regarding the recommended length of treatment; however, antidepressants are generally continued for at least six months and often a year for depressed people who are not alcoholic. This recommendation seems reasonable. If the alcoholic continues drinking or relapses from sobriety, medication often can be continued although compliance may become a significant problem. With sparse data to guide treatment, expect variation among physicians, who will likely rely, in part, on their own clinical experience.

Alcoholics with bipolar disorder (previously called manic-depressive disorder) are usually prescribed mood-stabilizing medications. A logical choice would be one of the anticonvulsants approved for bipolar disorder, and also demonstrated to help reduce alcohol abuse. Both divalproex sodium and carbamazepine are in this category. It is unknown whether topiramate is effective for bipolar disorder because the necessary studies have not been done. Some of the newer antipsychotic medications have been approved for bipolar disorder, but well-designed and controlled studies have not been conducted to evaluate either positive or negative effects on alcohol abuse.

Anxiety disorders are frequently present in alcoholics. It is not known whether these disorders exist prior to development of alcoholism, are co-occurring, or are even caused by prolonged alcohol use. Benzodiazepines are often prescribed for anxiety disorders (see above) but have risks of dangerous interactions with alcohol. Benzodiazepines are also known to cause physical and psychological dependence. While they are certainly less problematic than alcohol, benzodiazepines can become another addiction, and not a favorable outcome for alcoholics.

An alternative medication for anxiety is buspirone, marketed as Buspar®. Buspirone is not sedating, does not interact with alcohol, and does not appear to have risk for addiction or physical dependence. Unfortunately, it often requires several weeks to become effective, and few alcoholics can tolerate persistent anxiety for that long without relapse. Nevertheless, in the available studies, three of four well-designed studies indicated that buspirone can reduce alcohol consumption while reducing anxiety. Buspirone might be worth the effort required to use it effectively.

Something that works, providing ...

Don Goodwin recommended an approach to treating alcoholism which he believed worked every time, given one stipulation—the patient must do what the doctor says. In this case he must do only one thing: come to the office every three or four days.

As a rule, doctors cannot help patients who refuse to do what they say, and so there is nothing unusual about the stipulation. Why every three or four days? Because the effect of Antabuse® lasts up to five days after a person takes it. If the patient takes Antabuse® in the office, in the presence of the doctors, they both know that he will not drink for up to five days. They have bought time, a precious thing in the treatment of alcoholism.

This approach involves other things besides Antabuse®, but Antabuse® makes the other things possible. First, it gives hope, and hope by the time the alcoholic sees a doctor is often in short supply. He feels that his case is hopeless, his family feels that it is hopeless, and often the doctor feels that it is hopeless. With this approach the doctor can say, 'I can help you with your drinking problem' and mean it. He doesn't mean that he can help him forever (forever is a long time) and it doesn't mean that the patient won't still be unhappy or that he will become a new man. It merely means that he will not drink as long as he comes to the office every three or four days and takes the Antabuse®. Properly warned, he won't drink unless he is crazy or stupid, and if either is the case, he probably should not be given Antabuse®.

On the first visit the doctor can say something like this:

> Your problem, or at least your immediate problem, is that you have trouble controlling your drinking. Let me take charge; let me control your drinking for a time. This will be my responsibility. Come in, take the pill, and then we can deal with other things.

> I want you to stop drinking for a month. [At this point the doctor makes a note in his desk calendar to remind himself when the patient will have taken Antabuse® for a month.] After that we can discuss whether you want to continue taking the pill. It will be your decision.

> You need to stop for a month for two reasons. First, I need to know whether there is anything wrong with you besides drinking too much. You may have another problem that I can treat, such as a depression, but I won't be able to find out until you stop drinking for at least several weeks. Alcohol itself makes people depressed and anxious, and mimics all kinds of psychiatric illnesses.

> Secondly, I want you to stop drinking for a month to have a chance to see that life is bearable—sometimes just barely bearable—without alcohol. Millions of people don't drink and manage. You can manage too, but you haven't had a chance recently to discover this.

F. Scott Fitzgerald complained that he could never get sober long enough to tolerate sobriety, and at least this much can be achieved with the present approach.

It is important for the patient to see the doctor (or whatever professional is responsible for his care) whenever he comes for the pill. As a rule, patients want to please their doctors; this is probably why they are more punctual in keeping office appointments than doctors are in seeing them. In the beginning the patient may be coming, in part, as a kind of favor to the doctor.

The visits can be as brief or as long as time permits. The essential thing is that rapport be established, that the patient believes something is being done to help him, and that he stays on the wagon (he has no choice if he lives up to his part of the doctor–patient contract). Frequent brief visits can accomplish these things.

The emphasis during the visit should not be on the pill but on the problems most alcoholics face when they stop drinking. The major problem is finding out what to do with all the time that has suddenly become available now that drinking can no longer fill it. Boredom is the curse of the non-drinking drinking man. For years, most of the pleasurable things in his life have been associated with drinking: food, sex, companionship, fishing, Sunday-afternoon football. Without alcohol these things lose some of their attraction. The alcoholic tends to withdraw, brood, feel sorry for himself.

The therapist may help him to find substitute pleasure—hobbies, social activities not revolving around alcohol, anything that kills time and may give some satisfaction, if not anything as satisfying as a boozy glow. In time he may find these things for himself, but meanwhile life can be awfully monotonous.

Also, the patient can bring up problems of living that tend to accumulate when a person has drunk a lot. People usually feel better when they talk about problems, particularly when the listener is warm and friendly and doesn't butt into the conversation by talking about his own problems. The therapist can help by listening even if he cannot solve the problems.

If he is a mental health specialist, he can also do a thorough psychiatric examination, looking for something other than drinking to diagnose and treat. Not uncommonly, alcoholics turn out to have a depressive illness, phobias, or other psychiatric conditions.

One thing the therapist can do is to help the patient accept his alcoholism. This is sometimes difficult. Alcoholics have spent most of their drinking careers persuading themselves and others that they do not have a drinking problem. The habit of self-deception, set and hardened over so many years, is hard to break. William James describes this habit with his usual verve, and concludes that the alcoholic's salvation begins with breaking it.

How many excuses does the drunkard find when each new temptation comes! Others are drinking and it would be churlishness to refuse; or it is but to enable him to sleep, or just to get through this job of work; or it isn't drinking, it is because he feels so cold; or it is Christmas Day; or it is means of stimulating him to make a more powerful resolution in favor of abstinence than any he has hitherto made; or it is just this once, and once doesn't count … its, in fact, anything you like except being a drunkard. But if … through thick and thin he holds to it that he is a drunkard and nothing else, he is not likely to remain one long. The effort by which he succeeds in keeping the right name unwaveringly present to his mind proves to be his saving moral act.

William James

After a month of taking the pill and talking about problems, what happens then? The patient and doctor renegotiate. Almost invariably, the patient decides to take the pill for another month. The doctor says OK, and this is the first step in a process that must occur if the patient is going to recover: acceptance of personal responsibility for control of his drinking.

Proceeding on a month-to-month basis is a variation on the AA principle that an alcoholic should take each day as it comes.

For years, alcohol has been the most important thing in the alcoholic's life, or close to it. To be told that he can never drink again is about as depressing as anything he can hear. It may not even be true. Studies indicate that a small percentage of alcoholics return to 'normal' drinking for long periods. They tend to be on the low end of the continuum of severity, but not always. 'Controlled' drinking is probably a better term than 'normal' drinking, since alcoholics continue to invest alcohol with a significance that would never occur to the truly normal drinker.

Many people, especially some AA members, reject the notion that alcoholics can ever drink normally. If alcoholism is defined as a permanent inability to drink normally, then obviously any person about to drink normally for a long period was never an alcoholic in the first place. The issue is really one of definition, and those few alcoholics who reported sustained periods of controlled drinking in the studies were at any rate considered alcoholic when they weren't drinking normally. Most clinicians would agree that it is a mistake to encourage a severe classical alcoholic to believe he can ever again drink normally, but on the other hand telling him that he can never drink again seems unnecessary and may not be true in every case.

When does treatment end? The minimum period is one month because that is the basis for the doctor–patient contract agreed upon in advance. Ideally, however, the treatment should continue for a minimum of six months, with the patient himself making the decision to continue taking Antabuse® on a month-to-month basis. Why six months? Because there is evidence that most alcoholics who begin drinking again do so within the first six months following abstention.

A general rule applies here: the longer a patient goes without drinking at all, the shorter the relapse if a relapse occurs. It takes time to adapt to a sober way of life. Both the doctor and patient should be prepared for relapses. Alcoholism, by definition, is a chronic relapsing condition, although relapses are not inevitable. It resembles manic-depressive disease in this regard and also has similarities to such chronic medical illnesses as diabetes and multiple sclerosis. When the alcoholic has a relapse, his physician often feels resentful. When his diabetic patient has a relapse because he failed to take insulin, the doctor tends to be more understanding. The reason for this inconsistency is not clear.

Three objections have been raised concerning the above approach to treating alcoholism. The treatment is said to be based on fear, namely the fear of getting sick, and fear is held to be one of the least desirable forms of motivation. This is debatable. Fear may be the only reason that some alcoholics stop drinking. There is evidence that internists have somewhat better success in treating alcoholics than psychiatrists do, and the reason may be that they are in a better position to frighten the patient. They have merely to examine his liver and tell him he may be dead in a year if he keeps on drinking. Innumerable alcoholics have stopped drinking because they were told something like this. Others have stopped because they were afraid of losing their wives or their jobs. It is probably no coincidence that the hardest alcoholics to treat are those who have little to lose—those who have already lost their wives, jobs, and health. They have no hope of regaining these. All they have left to lose is their life, and, by now, living has little appeal. Probably the most effective alcoholism-treatment programs are run by industries, where the patient is an employee and his job depends on staying sober. The quotation at the beginning of this chapter is from Gorham's fictional study of an alcoholic, Carlotta McGride. As Gorham says, alcohol works. It has worked for the alcoholic for many years. Unless he is very much afraid of something, he probably will not give it up.

The second objection to the approach outlined here is that the patient becomes too dependent on a personal relationship with an authority figure, the physician, which must end at some point. In the treatment of alcoholism, the goal is not so much a lifetime cure (although sometimes this happens) as it is to bring about improvement. If the patient stays sober for longer periods after treatment than he did before, the treatment has been at least a limited success. In any case, the physician should discourage a dependent relationship. He can insist upon the patient taking the pill and staying dry for a month (realizing that a month is an arbitrary unit of time and any fixed interval will do), but after that the patient has to realize that he himself has the ultimate responsibility for the control of his drinking.

The issue of dependence on authority is particularly relevant for the UK where there is evidence that supervised Antabuse® is an effective treatment, especially when the supervisor is someone close to a patient, such as a spouse or friend. Turning over supervision to a person who actually lives with the patient is a great advantage. It reduces the number of office visits and also can be carried on for much longer than six months. Sometimes a 'contract' is signed by the therapist, patient, and supervisor. The supervisor may actually watch the patient take the Antabuse®, but this is not usually necessary. If the patient starts drinking again, obviously he has not been taking his pill. Standing over an adult and watching him take a pill may have an infantilizing effect on the patient and cause resentment—sometimes sufficient resentment to excuse more drinking. One useful clause in the contract (whether written or verbal) is that the wife promises never to mention her husband's previous drinking in any context as long as he continues taking the Antabuse®. The victims in the family—wife, husband, children—remember all the bad things that happen when the drinking member of the family was drunk. It tends to leave a lasting scar on the relationship. Many alcoholics are willing to take Antabuse® or do practically anything to stop the nagging and harping about past misbehavior.

Supervised Antabuse® is a much neglected treatment modality in countries other than the UK. It should be tried elsewhere. It often seems to work. Now, back to the 'American plan' of office supervision.

Finally, the complaint is heard that this approach does not get to the root of the problem—it does not explain how the patient became an alcoholic. This is true but, in our opinion, no one can explain how a person becomes an alcoholic because no one knows the cause of alcoholism. Doctors sometimes blame the patient's upbringing and patients often blame everyday stresses. There is no way to validate either explanation. There is probably no harm in telling the patient that his condition remains a medical mystery. And despite the evidence presented in Chapter 11, it is still premature to say that he inherited his disease.

However, if it is ever shown conclusively that some forms of alcoholism are influenced by heredity, this would not make the prognosis less favorable or the treatment less helpful. Sometimes, when evidence for a genetic factor is presented, you hear the following: 'But if it is genetic, then you can't do anything about it'. It should be noted that adult-onset diabetes is almost certainly a genetic disorder and there are excellent treatments for diabetes.

17

Alcoholics Anonymous (AA)

> ... Drop the anvil!
>
> AA joke (see p. 149)

Since its creation in 1935 by two alcoholics, AA has grown into a worldwide network of self-help services for alcoholics and their families. It continues to dominate alcoholism treatment in the USA, in hospital settings as well as church basements; it has fared less well in other countries, particularly in Russia and the Orient.

AA has many attractive features, including the common denominators of psychotherapy and—at no cost—the assurance of a regular sympathetic hearing, the feeling that somebody is taking one's condition seriously, the discovery that others are in the same predicament. Unlike most talking therapies, AA expends little effort on trying to explain why anyone is alcoholic. The term 'allergy' is sometimes used, but usually properly bracketed in quotation marks (alcoholism does not, of course, resemble conventional allergies at all).

There is an old idea that alcoholics must become religious in order to stop drinking, and it is true that AA has certain similarities to a religion and that some of its members have been 'converted' to AA in the same way they would be to other religions. Its 'twelve steps', for example, have a definite religious flavor, emphasizing a reliance on a higher power, usually assumed to be God, the need for forgiveness, and caring for others. Alcoholics vary in expression of the personal characteristic of spirituality and faith (as does the rest of the population). A recent study found that alcoholics who are not interested in religion or spirituality had less attendance or benefit from AA. Insisting that uninterested alcoholics attend AA, which has long been a treatment mainstay, may result in more frustration than recovery.

Nevertheless, to the extent that it is a religion, AA is one of the least doctrinaire and authoritarian religions imaginable. Atheists can belong to AA as comfortably as believers. There is no formal doctrine and no insistence that anyone accept a particular explanation for alcoholism. AA gives drinkers something to do when they are not drinking. It offers occasions for the soul-satisfying experience of helping someone else. It provides companions who do not drink. And it provides hope for those who need it desperately—the alcoholic and his family—and instant help for the person who wants to get back on the wagon and can't quite make it.

This sounds like a wonderful package of services, and AA is often credited with helping more alcoholics than all other alcoholism treatments combined. There is no way of knowing whether this is true, since the kind of careful studies needed to prove this point have not been done. However, most professionals working with alcoholics agree that certainly nothing is lost by encouraging them to attend AA meetings, and possibly much can be gained.

How does an alcoholic arrive at this first AA meeting? There are several routes. In despair, alone or at the urging of family or friends, he may call the number in the phone book, locate a meeting, and go by himself or be escorted. His doctor or clergyman may suggest it. He may be visited by an AA member in a hospital or prison, perhaps going to his meeting in the institution.

> When he arrives, he is likely to be frightened, depressed and still sick from withdrawal after his last drink
>
> writes Margaret Bean in her book *Alcoholics Anonymous*. It was written in 1975, but matters have not changed much since then.
>
> If he comes on his own and speaks to no one, he will probably be left alone. If he approaches someone or asks for help, however, he will almost invariably get it. Most people, at first, treat him with reserve, friendly interest, and encouragement. The usual practice is for the veteran member to talk about his drinking problem but not push the newcomer to reveal his. Most members realize that the newcomer has lost his self-esteem, is overcome with guilt and remorse, and feels that his weakness is all too apparent. They do not expect him to reciprocate confessional stories. The initial transaction is the instillation of hope.
>
> The new member is taken under the wing of some sympathetic person as a 'pigeon', or beginner. He is asked if he has admitted to himself that he has trouble with alcohol, and whether he has accepted his problem. 'Admitting' and 'accepting' are carefully distinguished as separate steps. He is urged to

come to many meetings, preferably '90 meetings in 90 days', because as a newcomer he needs them. He is taught that he should listen, keep his opinions to himself, ask questions when he does not understand, and observe and imitate successful members. He often is encouraged to give up all social contacts outside AA. The express reason for this is that he is in danger from them, because they were where he 'caught' alcoholism in the first place.

While a new member is not pushed to disclose details about himself, it is suggested that it would do him good to find someone he can talk with about his drinking. The idea is that he will find it a relief to confess all the things of which he is ashamed. For some AA members, AA may totally replace non-AA social activities.

All AA groups provide members with a protected environment in which they are treated as equal, regardless of the extent of their alcohol problem. They are freed from the fear that besets new relationships in conventional society, that one's alcoholic history will be discovered and one will be rejected because of it.

Long sobriety does confer status in AA, but there are safeguards against holier-than-thou attitudes, since at some point all members were stigmatized as alcoholics and no one is in a position to point an accusing finger ...

Recovery is divided into three stages—physical, emotional, and spiritual. Physical recovery is the first step and the one in which Twelve Steppers are most active in the AA outreach system. A call comes for help from someone who is still sobering up. A worker at Central Service will talk with him on the telephone for a while or contact a member on call for Twelve Step work and make immediate personal contact.

The Twelve Step worker usually gets a new member to a meeting within 24 hours if possible. He knows that the desire to drink is very strong in the early stages of physical recovery and encourages the newcomer to go to as many meetings as possible.

Meetings are either open—anyone who wants to come is welcome—or closed to non-alcoholics. A new member usually has a sponsor, the person in whom he chooses to confide early in his membership. All AA meetings accept any alcoholic; some AA groups may focus on particular interests or characteristics, such as gays, lesbians, men or women, professionals, bikers, physicians and health-care providers, etc. The goal of AA is total abstinence, and the idea of controlled drinking is strongly discouraged.

Many AA members go to meetings with each other, see each other relapse and return, watch each other stay sober longer and longer. Many apparently expect to continue to do so several nights a week for the rest of their lives. Sometimes their families sabotage them in their use of AA and sometimes support them. Most often they are deeply loyal and very grateful to AA.

Alcoholics Anonymous

Margaret Bean

AA has two 'bibles'. One is called *Twelve Steps and Twelve Traditions*. The other is named *Alcoholics Anonymous*, called the 'Big Book' by members. The latter is a volume of anecdotal accounts of experiences with alcohol written by early members. The *Twelve Traditions* book describes the organization itself. It stresses that AA is not a reform movement, nor is it operated by professionals. It is financed by voluntary contributions from its members, all of whom remain anonymous. There are no dues, no paid therapist. All comers who want help are accepted as members. All groups are autonomous. AA does not endorse other enterprises or take sides in controversies. (AA has learned a lesson from the Washington Society, a self-help group of alcoholics in the mid-nineteenth century that floundered on internal dissent over antislavery and other issues.)

When Bill W, co-founder of AA, was asked earnestly, 'How does AA work?' he was fond of answering, 'Just fine, thanks. Just fine'. Three chapters in the Big Book (Chapters 5–7) explain how AA works in detail. These are devoted essentially to the 'twelve suggested steps of recovery'.

The Twelve Steps

1. We admitted we were powerless over alcohol—that our lives had become unmanageable.

2. Came to believe that a Power greater than ourselves could restore us to sanity.

3. Made a decision to turn our will and our lives over to the care of God as we understand Him.

4. Made a searching and fearless moral inventory of our lives.

5. Admitted to God, to ourselves, and to another human being the exact nature of our wrongs.

6. Were entirely ready to have God remove all these defects of character.

7. Humbly asked Him to remove our shortcomings.

8. Made a list of all persons we had harmed, and became willing to make amends to them all.

9. Made direct amends to such people wherever possible.

10. Continued to take personal inventory and when we were wrong promptly admitted it.

11. Sought through prayer and meditation to improve our conscious contact with God as we understood him, praying only for knowledge of His will for us and the power to carry that out.

12. Having had a spiritual awakening as the result of these steps, we tried to carry this message to alcoholics and to practise these principles in all our affairs.

Note that only two of the twelve steps mention alcohol. More than a prescription of abstinence, the step gives a prescription for living.

As one AA member stated,

AA doesn't teach us how to handle our drinking; it teaches us to handle sobriety. Most of us knew before we came through the door of the first meeting that the way to handle our drinking was to quit. People told us so. Almost every alcoholic I know has stopped drinking at one time or another—maybe dozens of times! So it is no trick to stop drinking; the trick is how to stay stopped.

Many AA members approach twelve-step 'work' with an open mind and are prepared to be flexible. 'Greater Power', for many, stands for AA itself. God may be a symbol for the mystery of the universe rather than a traditional deity.

How successful is AA?

Some years ago, the Rand Corporation in the USA completed the most extensive study of alcoholism ever made at that time. Information was obtained on 85 per cent of 922 men who had received treatment in an alcoholism unit. They were followed over four years. The report found that alcoholics who regularly attended AA had a higher rate of long-term abstinence than all the other groups. About half were abstinent after four years. However, only 14 percent of the patients were regularly attending AA at the end of four years. Patients had not been randomly assigned to AA groups and other forms of treatment. Conceivably, the small minority regularly attending AA after four years represented a highly motivated group that would have done as well receiving some other treatment or no treatment.

Systematic and replicable research is very difficult with AA: the organization maintains principles of autonomy of groups and individuals, and thus does not mandate participation in any research; alcoholics self-select different groups, thus preventing generalizing to a larger population; and is it not possible to change the content or structure of the twelve steps to determine what elements are necessary for success. More recently, some studies have attempted to determine whether a therapy method of introducing alcoholics to AA might be useful. The best example is from the MATCH study, which was a large multicenter study of the effect of customizing alcoholism treatment to individual needs. This study found that engendering active participation in AA was as effective in maintaining abstinence as two other therapy methods, cognitive-behavioral therapy and motivational enhancement. Considering the role of AA in most treatment programs and recommendations, it is unfortunate that more research has not been undertaken.

The fact remains that AA has received higher praise from more people than any other approach to the problem.

> In view of the fact that all speakers adhere to a formula and everyone knows how it is going to turn out, meetings are surprisingly varied and entertaining. Speakers vary in education, charm, articulateness, age, and sex. Each tells a story: How he started to drink, lost control, and began to destroy everything in his life that had been important to him. Each has his own version of hitting bottom and —despairing, disbelieving, and full of revulsion and uncertainty—coming to AA. He then describes his recovery and how he has been able to cope with his life without alcohol.
>
> *Alcoholics Anonymous*
> Margaret Bean

An AA member came to our medical school to talk with students. Her story gives the flavor of AA meetings around the world and passes on some good advice to young doctors-to-be.

ⓘ Patient's perspective

Hi, I'm Carol—I am an alcoholic. This is the way we introduce ourselves in an AA meeting and it seems appropriate to begin that way.

To begin with the vital statisticals. I have been married to a professional man for 25 years. We have three sons. I have been sober for two and one-half years. I am a registered nurse. During the period of the alcoholism I was attending the university where I earned a bachelor's degree in sociology. After I became sober I returned to school and this semester I will finish a master's degree in social work. I plan to work in the field of alcoholism when I graduate.

My life before the age of 38 was wholly unremarkable. There is no alcoholism in my immediate family, but my paternal grandfather was clearly alcoholic. My parents had a stable marriage; I was neither neglected nor abused as a child. I had what one could consider a normal adolescence, I had no problem with authority, and made straight As in school. I was socialized to be a wife and mother; my nursing degree was strictly an insurance policy, not a career. It should be clear I was raised before the women's movement. It was a search for my own identity that precipitated the crisis leading to the alcoholism. Those of you who have seen the movie *Kramer vs. Kramer* can have some idea of how I lapsed into dysfunction. Except that I lacked that woman's courage to confront the problem directly and took the back door out into depression and alcoholism.

When I became depressed I didn't understand what was happening to me. I only knew that I was miserable and that there was something terribly wrong with me. I went to see a psychiatrist who started giving me antidepressants and tranquilizers. I took those drugs almost constantly until I entered an alcoholism treatment center where they took me off cold turkey and I went through withdrawal. I saw the psychiatrist on a weekly basis except when he was on vacation or I was. At the end of four and one-half years of traditional psychotherapy and drugs I was still depressed, alcoholic, and addicted to those drugs as well.

It is always difficult for an alcoholic to identify that moment in time when you cross from normal to alcoholic drinking. I can see now that I was getting into trouble when I began using alcohol as medicine. I began to drink at bedtime to combat the insomnia that plagued me. I drank a lot to quell the fear and anxiety that overwhelmed me. The longer I drank, the greater the anxiety grew—a connection I was unable to make at the time. I also drank for all the reasons everyone else drinks—because I thought it made me feel better; any occasion seems more festive if you drink. I drank a lot to gain confidence in myself—something that has never been my long suit. I also used Librium for that purpose and I can tell you that in my drugged days this would be at least a 100 mg performance.

Let me establish my credentials by telling you that before I began my recovery I was hospitalized twice for detoxification, I made a serious attempt at suicide, I left my husband at one point, only to have the drinking grow even worse, and I returned. I suffered innumerable blackouts. The longest blackout I had lasted for 24 hours. I woke up on Thursday to find out it was Friday. I used to park my car in a blackout when I went to class and then couldn't find it when I came out. I hid bottles all over the house, and sometimes did that in a blackout and couldn't find them later. During the first year of my sobriety they kept turning up all over the house.

I was a binge drinker. I would have a period of weeks of sobriety or social drinking followed by several days of uncontrolled drinking. The binges grew closer and closer together. My husband learned to time them and could often tell when he could expect to return home and find me drinking again. During this time I was trying to stay sober on will power. My psychiatrist gave me Antabuse, but it didn't do any good. Usually when I found it necessary to drink again I realized I had conveniently forgotten to take the Antabuse. And then I made the dangerous discovery that I could drink within two days of stopping the Antabuse and the reaction was tolerable. Toward the end my psychiatrist tried to get me to go to AA, but I refused. Someone might see me and suspect that I was an alcoholic—and that would have been the absolute end of the world! Besides, I kept asking, what could a bunch of ex-drunks do for me that a board-certified psychiatrist could not? The only thing my doctor told me was that it would give me someone to call in case I wanted to take a drink.

The turning point came when my husband came to the end of his rope. He sat me down for another of our many talks where we would both agree that I simply had to stop drinking and I would go out again and try it on will power. Only this time it was different—this time he was telling me what he was going to do: 'Alcohol is controlling your life and therefore it is controlling mine and I won't have it'. In desperation he turned to a friend of ours who is a nurse and she had found out about treatment centers and had gotten him some Al-Anon literature. My doctor had never told him about the organization. My husband tried to get me to go for treatment but I did not want to go to a mental institution, so I threw myself on his mercy with pitiful tears and pleading—something that I was very good at doing. He gave in, but extracted a promise that if I took one more drink I would go to treatment. The week had not ended until I was drinking again and he carted me off to a treatment center. I tried to leave after I got there and he told me if I came home I would go back with a sheriff because he would commit me. Out of the fog of the final days of my drinking I can recall the expression on the faces of my family and psychiatrist. It was a look of infinite sadness. As though they were saying to themselves: 'She was such a nice person—too bad she's lost'. It was like being present at my own funeral. Their attitude reinforced my own feeling of hopelessness.

In forcing me into treatment my husband provided that last final ingredient for recovery from alcoholism—and that is hope. For the first time in my life I met recovering alcoholics and learned about AA. My behavior was perfectly understandable to them. I was an alcoholic. They seemed to know without my telling them all the helplessness, hopelessness, fear, and anger that raged inside me. And because they understood me so thoroughly I began to believe that perhaps what had worked for them could work for me as well.

There is a spiritual component to recovery from alcoholism. It is that moment of truth when the alcoholic says, 'I give up. I surrender. I will do anything to stop drinking and change my life'. This is commonly known as 'hitting bottom'. It is a very painful experience for the alcoholic. For now he must give up all the defenses that have been protecting him from painful reality. You feel like you're standing naked before the whole world.

Those of us who recover in AA believe that a part of this surrender is a willingness to accept belief in a Power Greater Than Ourselves, whatever one conceives that to be. For me this occurred during the second week of my recovery. I was experiencing acute withdrawal from the Librium and I was virtually paralyzed with anxiety. I was terrified that I was losing my mind and would spend the rest of my life in a mental institution. And in that, the lowest ebb of my life, I got in touch with the infinitude of my being. I gave up intellectualizing about who or what God might or might not be and prayer welled up from inside me, a simple 'Help me—for I cannot help myself'. And when I reached out, help was there for me in the form of the AA program and all the alcoholics who so lovingly taught me how to put it into practice in my own life.

I was in treatment for five weeks. When I returned home I was terrified that I would slip back in to my old behavior pattern and start drinking again. But I attended AA regularly and tried diligently to work the program. And one day at a time I managed to stay sober. And the days lengthened into weeks and then into months and the day came that I realized that I not only hadn't taken a drink that day—I hadn't even thought about taking a drink. The obsession was leaving me. I can't tell you what an enormous sense of relief I felt when I finally realized I don't ever have to drink again.

And then I came to realize that I was experiencing life differently than I ever had before. As I have come to recognize the changes in my behavior and attitudes, I have realized that without the pain of the alcoholism I would never have opened myself up to the possibility of growth. I could have muddled around in depression and self-pity for the rest of my life if the alcoholism had not forced me to deal with it. Sometimes in AA meetings you hear an alcoholic say, 'I thank God I am an alcoholic'. The first time I heard that I hadn't been sober very long and I thought they must have been brain damaged. But I understand now what he is saying. You also sometimes hear alcoholics say, 'I had to do everything I did to be where I am today'. That is for me the epitome of self-acceptance.

I want to take a few minutes to speak to you briefly about your own attitudes toward alcoholism. The medical profession taught me that alcoholics are hopeless. As a student nurse I hated alcoholic patients. They tried my patience when they were admitted drunk and took up my time that I felt better spent on patients whom I considered to be really sick. I learned this attitude from the doctors and nurses who taught me. A doctor who was teaching us said: 'I want to warn you girls about the alcoholics you will be taking care of on the wards. They can charm your socks off, but don't you be fooled—you can never get an alcoholic to stay sober'. In those days I believed everything doctors told me—I was to learn better much later. But in any case I had no reason to doubt him. I never saw anyone get sober either.

And so I ask you to stay very closely in touch with your attitudes as you begin to practice medicine. If you think alcoholism is a moral problem, then you won't be inclined to intervene very actively in the disease process.

By a moral problem I mean if you think the alcoholic can quit drinking by himself using will power, if he will only get his act together.

I believe alcoholism is a disease in the sense that it is something that happens to you—just as cancer or heart disease happens to you. I did not ask to become alcoholic. That was never one of my goals in life. But I was forced back into contact with reality one day and realized that I had become the victim of a process with a known symptomatology, a predictable course, and a terrible prognosis. That process is called alcoholism.

We don't know what causes it, but not knowing what causes a disease has never before stopped the medical profession from treating it. I am reminded of a joke you sometimes hear around AA meetings. This drunk wanders down to the edge of a lake carrying an anvil. He's going to swim across to the other side. He jumps in and very soon he's drowning. Now on the opposite shore are all these people who want to help him. The ministers are yelling, 'We're praying for you, we're praying for you'. The doctors are yelling, 'We're doing research, we're doing research'. The AA members are yelling, 'DROP THE ANVIL!'

18

Attacking the problem

Prevention of alcoholism is an impossible dream, people say, and maybe they are right. Fifty years ago the prevention of polio was an impossible dream. People said it, and they were wrong. Twenty years ago, AIDS was thought to be virtually untreatable and fatal, yet now medication may prolong life for decades and prevention efforts have slowed the epidemic spread of the disease in some places. It is true that the prevention of alcoholism is still at the 'safe sex and clean needle' stage, but it may not always be that way.

What can any of us—the family, employer, doctor, or society—do to help prevent alcoholism or arrest it at an early stage?

What can the family do?

First, it can recognize the problem when there is one. There often is great reluctance to do so. Alcoholism is not a socially acceptable disease; there is no straight-forward cure, and many people still believe that the alcoholic chooses to misbehave. First the problem has to be seen as a problem—but then what?

Nothing is more frustrating for someone in the helping business (doctor, social worker, etc.) than to get a call from a spouse: 'John is drinking too much. What can I do?'

'Well have him come see me.'

'But he won't. He doesn't think he has a drinking problem. I'm desperate. What should I do?'

Call the police? What can the police do? Usually nothing. Drinking is not a crime. Wife-beating is, and that is when the police may help (but usually not help with the drinking).

Nag? Nagging just provides another reason to drink.

Threaten? Well, yes, sometimes. If the last straw is really the last straw, it is probably a good idea to say so. Sometimes people do stop drinking because a husband or wife threatens to leave them. Coercion sometimes works. However, often it isn't the last straw, but next to the last straw, and what then? If threats or importuning don't work, what will?

Family life poses few problems as painful as this one. How the spouse handles it says a good deal about the spouse and the nature of the relationship. In their own ways, husbands and wives play out the roles society and their own unique personalities assign to them, and usually there is not as much 'choice' as people like to believe. Advice, even from the wisest adviser, may be bad advice simply because family relations are tremendously complicated, played out intuitively by and large, and outsiders never know how it really is.

Advice to be tender or tough (to leave him or not) is usually best not given, and most people don't listen anyway.

Some general principles

◆ Violent behavior in a drunk person is frightening to witness, especially for children, and can be very dangerous. The spouse should first and foremost protect themselves and their children by going to a neighbor or relative's house, or other refuge. Any efforts to discuss the behavior should be reserved for a time when the drinker is sober and willing to speak rationally.

◆ The alcoholic must face the consequences of his behavior. The family often tries to protect him from these consequences and shouldn't. Don't pick up the pieces. If he passes out leave him there. If he throws up, let him clean it up the next morning. If he doesn't remember how the window was broken, tell him later. Be matter of fact. Don't pretend it was funny.

◆ Don't say I told you so. (Blackouts are scary. Sometimes people stop drinking because of them. Don't let him forget he forgot.)

◆ Don't buy him a drink.

◆ Don't call the boss to say he has the flu (a hard rule to follow when the family depends on the income).

◆ Don't bail him out of jail—or anything else. Let him explain—not you. Let him apologize—not you.

> ◆ Stop trying to control his drinking behavior. You can't anyway. You are as powerless in this regard as he is. Stop playing games. Stop hiding bottles. Stop pouring them down drains. Stop organizing the family routine around his drinking. Stop babying him. Allow him to be responsible for his behavior. Love the sinner but not the sin.

Help is available. AA has an excellent website currently posted in three different languages: English, Spanish, and French. The site contains basic information about the program, and how to obtain program material and services for members. You can find meeting locations and times in each of the 51 US states and Canada. You can also identify AA General Service Offices in 59 different countries around the world. If you aren't particularly computer savvy, most local telephone directories will have a listing for AA. Alanon (support for friends and families of alcoholics) and Alateen (support for teenagers affected by problem drinkers) also have Internet support services with chat lines, meeting listings, and international links. The website for the National Council on Alcohol and Drug Dependence can also direct you to various service groups in the USA.

AA usually won't send someone to your house unless they are invited by the alcoholic, but the spouse can go to Alanon and the children can go to Alateen. These organizations may be the best first step towards identifying resources and deciding on a course of action.

There is reason for hope

Much has changed over the years since *Alcoholism: the facts* first went into print in 1981. Many more resources exist to help alcoholics and their families today than ever before. Scientists have a much better understanding of the problem. They are only beginning to unravel the many complicated psychological, biochemical, and physiological dimensions that make up the disease. And they are finally beginning to develop useful strategies to combat it. For the first time in history, meaningful treatment options are available that do help. They only help. They do not cure, but it is a start.

Physicians are called upon to do more. Studies show that brief 'bedside' interventions do help. The National Institute on Alcohol Abuse and Alcoholism website contains brief screening instruments and interventions with scripts to help doctors find the right words. Many of the new medications are also easily managed by primary care physicians. Doctors can make a difference. And alcoholics need them to try.

Society is called upon to set aside its frustration and moral judgments of the drinker, and to redefine its roles and attitudes toward drinking. Alcoholics do need to be held accountable for their actions, but they are entitled to a measure of compassion. Society should also avoid being an inadvertent accomplice in the development of drinking problems through the promotion and glamorization of reckless alcohol use. Better education programs are still needed to reach those who are at risk. This is especially important for the young drinker; so that any problems may be addressed early.

The treatment community no longer clings to the 'quit drinking or die' philosophy. The future of the alcoholic does not have to be so bleak. Alcoholism is increasingly recognized as a chronic lifelong disease. It is understood that slips can and do occur, even after many years of success. But with commitment and hard work many alcoholics do recover and can live normal productive and fulfilling lives. That said, it is still important to recognize that, at least for now, the fight belongs to the alcoholic alone. No one, no family member or friend, can fight it for them. The alcoholic must accept the seriousness of their condition and commit fully to the process of recovery. If they are willing to do this, there is help for them. There is hope for the future.

Anne Lamott, a writer, a liberal, a Christian convert, and an alcoholic said this:

Hope begins in the dark, stubborn hope that if you just show up and try to do the right thing, the dawn will come. You wait and watch and work. You don't give up.

Notes

Chapter 1

1. Wood alcohol is composed of methanol, a one-carbon alcohol, which is metabolized by the body to formaldehyde and then formic acid. Drinking large amounts of methanol in a short time causes formic acid to build up and the pH of the blood to drop. It is the drop in blood pH that causes the symptoms associated with wood alcohol poisoning, such as blindness.

Chapter 2

1. Enzymes are biological molecules that are typically composed of one or more proteins. They act as biological catalysts, increasing the rate of biochemical reactions.

2. Hypogonadism is a condition characterized by inadequate or impaired function of the testes in males or ovaries in females.

Chapter 3

1. Oprah Winfrey is a popular American television talk show host.

Chapter 4

1. HDL and LDL refer to carrier molecules composed of fat and protein (i.e. lipoprotein) which escort the cholesterol molecule through the body. High-density lipoproteins transport cholesterol to the bile system for excretion from the body, whereas low-density lipoproteins carry cholesterol throughout the body via the bloodstream where it may accumulate on blood vessel walls.

Chapter 6

1. *Helicobacter pylori* is a type of bacterium which can infect the digestive system and damage its protective lining. *Helicobacter pylori* infection is believed to be responsible for the occurrence of a large proportion of peptic ulcers. Approximately 20 percent of adults under the age of 40 are infected; although most do not develop ulcers.

2. *Lunar caustic* appeared in the *Paris Review* in the Winter–Spring issue of 1963.

Chapter 8

1. The first British book on the subject, *Women and Alcohol*, was published in the autumn of 1980 by the Camberwell Council on Alcoholism. It holds that alcoholism among British women is indeed increasing, based on the following types of evidence. Since 1964 the number of men admitted to psychiatric hospitals in England and Wales with a diagnosis of alcoholism doubled; the corresponding number of women so diagnosed trebled. There was also a disproportionate increase in women's rates of convictions for drunkenness (including drunken driving), and for cirrhosis deaths and other forms of alcohol-related mortality. Agencies providing help for problem drinkers recorded a steady increase in women clients. This may seem persuasive, but increases in treatment cases and arrests do not necessarily mean an increase in the population. In recent years, alcoholism has become increasingly de-stigmatized and more alcoholics of both sexes are 'surfacing' in treatment facilities. Moreover, more treatment facilities exist, and there tends to be a correlation between opportunities for treatment and the number of people who seek treatment. To repeat, there is no direct evidence of an increase in female alcoholism.

2. Studies in animals and humans have linked FASD with abnormalities in the formation of glial cells, a type of neural support cell, especially in the brainstem and cerebellum. Specific structural abnormalities have also been identified in the corpus callosum.

Chapter 9

1. The adolescent brain is actively engaged in the remodeling of neural pathways (scientists call this *plasticity*). This activity enables them rapidly to adapt their neural connections to incorporate new experiences.

Chapter 11

1. Small protein molecules which may act as neurotransmitters.

Chapter 12

1. Positive reinforcement is a behavioral term for the selective strengthening of certain behaviors by the administration of a pleasurable stimulus or 'reward'.

Chapter 14

1. The term 'recovered' alcoholic deserves comment. AA takes the view that no one recovers from alcoholism; they simply stop drinking. Whether or not this is always the case, one should be cautioned against using terms that seem synonymous with 'recovered' but have different connotations. Terms to be avoided are 'ex-alcoholic' and 'reformed' alcoholic, as both have a criminalistic flavor.

Index